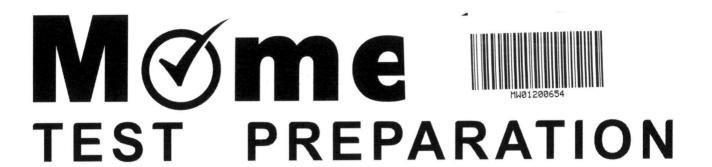

Mome
TEST PREPARATION

Trauma Certified Registered Nurse (TCRN)
Exam Secrets
Study Guide

DEAR FUTURE EXAM SUCCESS STORY

First of all, **THANK YOU** for purchasing Mometrix study materials!

Second, congratulations! You are one of the few determined test-takers who are committed to doing whatever it takes to excel on your exam. **You have come to the right place.** We developed these study materials with one goal in mind: to deliver you the information you need in a format that's concise and easy to use.

In addition to optimizing your guide for the content of the test, we've outlined our recommended steps for breaking down the preparation process into small, attainable goals so you can make sure you stay on track.

We've also analyzed the entire test-taking process, identifying the most common pitfalls and showing how you can overcome them and be ready for any curveball the test throws you.

Standardized testing is one of the biggest obstacles on your road to success, which only increases the importance of doing well in the high-pressure, high-stakes environment of test day. Your results on this test could have a significant impact on your future, and this guide provides the information and practical advice to help you achieve your full potential on test day.

Your success is our success

We would love to hear from you! If you would like to share the story of your exam success or if you have any questions or comments in regard to our products, please contact us at **800-673-8175** or **support@mometrix.com**.

Thanks again for your business and we wish you continued success!

Sincerely,
The Mometrix Test Preparation Team

> **Need more help? Check out our flashcards at:**
> **http://MometrixFlashcards.com/TCRN**

TABLE OF CONTENTS

Introduction

Thank you for purchasing this resource! You have made the choice to prepare yourself for a test that could have a huge impact on your future, and this guide is designed to help you be fully ready for test day. Obviously, it's important to have a solid understanding of the test material, but you also need to be prepared for the unique environment and stressors of the test, so that you can perform to the best of your abilities.

For this purpose, the first section that appears in this guide is the **Secret Keys**. We've devoted countless hours to meticulously researching what works and what doesn't, and we've boiled down our findings to the five most impactful steps you can take to improve your performance on the test. We start at the beginning with study planning and move through the preparation process, all the way to the testing strategies that will help you get the most out of what you know when you're finally sitting in front of the test.

We recommend that you start preparing for your test as far in advance as possible. However, if you've bought this guide as a last-minute study resource and only have a few days before your test, we recommend that you skip over the first two Secret Keys since they address a long-term study plan.

If you struggle with **test anxiety**, we strongly encourage you to check out our recommendations for how you can overcome it. Test anxiety is a formidable foe, but it can be beaten, and we want to make sure you have the tools you need to defeat it.

Secret Key #1 – Plan Big, Study Small

There's a lot riding on your performance. If you want to ace this test, you're going to need to keep your skills sharp and the material fresh in your mind. You need a plan that lets you review everything you need to know while still fitting in your schedule. We'll break this strategy down into three categories.

Information Organization

Start with the information you already have: the official test outline. From this, you can make a complete list of all the concepts you need to cover before the test. Organize these concepts into groups that can be studied together, and create a list of any related vocabulary you need to learn so you can brush up on any difficult terms. You'll want to keep this vocabulary list handy once you actually start studying since you may need to add to it along the way.

Time Management

Once you have your set of study concepts, decide how to spread them out over the time you have left before the test. Break your study plan into small, clear goals so you have a manageable task for each day and know exactly what you're doing. Then just focus on one small step at a time. When you manage your time this way, you don't need to spend hours at a time studying. Studying a small block of content for a short period each day helps you retain information better and avoid stressing over how much you have left to do. You can relax knowing that you have a plan to cover everything in time. In order for this strategy to be effective though, you have to start studying early and stick to your schedule. Avoid the exhaustion and futility that comes from last-minute cramming!

Study Environment

The environment you study in has a big impact on your learning. Studying in a coffee shop, while probably more enjoyable, is not likely to be as fruitful as studying in a quiet room. It's important to keep distractions to a minimum. You're only planning to study for a short block of time, so make the most of it. Don't pause to check your phone or get up to find a snack. It's also important to **avoid multitasking**. Research has consistently shown that multitasking will make your studying dramatically less effective. Your study area should also be comfortable and well-lit so you don't have the distraction of straining your eyes or sitting on an uncomfortable chair.

 The time of day you study is also important. You want to be rested and alert. Don't wait until just before bedtime. Study when you'll be most likely to comprehend and remember. Even better, if you know what time of day your test will be, set that time aside for study. That way your brain will be used to working on that subject at that specific time and you'll have a better chance of recalling information.

Finally, it can be helpful to team up with others who are studying for the same test. Your actual studying should be done in as isolated an environment as possible, but the work of organizing the information and setting up the study plan can be divided up. In between study sessions, you can discuss with your teammates the concepts that you're all studying and quiz each other on the details. Just be sure that your teammates are as serious about the test as you are. If you find that your study time is being replaced with social time, you might need to find a new team.

2

Secret Key #2 – Make Your Studying Count

You're devoting a lot of time and effort to preparing for this test, so you want to be absolutely certain it will pay off. This means doing more than just reading the content and hoping you can remember it on test day. It's important to make every minute of study count. There are two main areas you can focus on to make your studying count.

Retention

It doesn't matter how much time you study if you can't remember the material. You need to make sure you are retaining the concepts. To check your retention of the information you're learning, try recalling it at later times with minimal prompting. Try carrying around flashcards and glance at one or two from time to time or ask a friend who's also studying for the test to quiz you.

To enhance your retention, look for ways to put the information into practice so that you can apply it rather than simply recalling it. If you're using the information in practical ways, it will be much easier to remember. Similarly, it helps to solidify a concept in your mind if you're not only reading it to yourself but also explaining it to someone else. Ask a friend to let you teach them about a concept you're a little shaky on (or speak aloud to an imaginary audience if necessary). As you try to summarize, define, give examples, and answer your friend's questions, you'll understand the concepts better and they will stay with you longer. Finally, step back for a big picture view and ask yourself how each piece of information fits with the whole subject. When you link the different concepts together and see them working together as a whole, it's easier to remember the individual components.

Finally, practice showing your work on any multi-step problems, even if you're just studying. Writing out each step you take to solve a problem will help solidify the process in your mind, and you'll be more likely to remember it during the test.

Modality

Modality simply refers to the means or method by which you study. Choosing a study modality that fits your own individual learning style is crucial. No two people learn best in exactly the same way, so it's important to know your strengths and use them to your advantage.

For example, if you learn best by visualization, focus on visualizing a concept in your mind and draw an image or a diagram. Try color-coding your notes, illustrating them, or creating symbols that will trigger your mind to recall a learned concept. If you learn best by hearing or discussing information, find a study partner who learns the same way or read aloud to yourself. Think about how to put the information in your own words. Imagine that you are giving a lecture on the topic and record yourself so you can listen to it later.

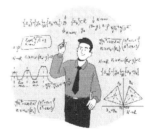

For any learning style, flashcards can be helpful. Organize the information so you can take advantage of spare moments to review. Underline key words or phrases. Use different colors for different categories. Mnemonic devices (such as creating a short list in which every item starts with the same letter) can also help with retention. Find what works best for you and use it to store the information in your mind most effectively and easily.

Secret Key #3 – Practice the Right Way

Your success on test day depends not only on how many hours you put into preparing, but also on whether you prepared the right way. It's good to check along the way to see if your studying is paying off. One of the most effective ways to do this is by taking practice tests to evaluate your progress. Practice tests are useful because they show exactly where you need to improve. Every time you take a practice test, pay special attention to these three groups of questions:

- The questions you got wrong
- The questions you had to guess on, even if you guessed right
- The questions you found difficult or slow to work through

This will show you exactly what your weak areas are, and where you need to devote more study time. Ask yourself why each of these questions gave you trouble. Was it because you didn't understand the material? Was it because you didn't remember the vocabulary? Do you need more repetitions on this type of question to build speed and confidence? Dig into those questions and figure out how you can strengthen your weak areas as you go back to review the material.

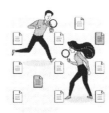 Additionally, many practice tests have a section explaining the answer choices. It can be tempting to read the explanation and think that you now have a good understanding of the concept. However, an explanation likely only covers part of the question's broader context. Even if the explanation makes perfect sense, **go back and investigate** every concept related to the question until you're positive you have a thorough understanding.

As you go along, keep in mind that the practice test is just that: practice. Memorizing these questions and answers will not be very helpful on the actual test because it is unlikely to have any of the same exact questions. If you only know the right answers to the sample questions, you won't be prepared for the real thing. **Study the concepts** until you understand them fully, and then you'll be able to answer any question that shows up on the test.

It's important to wait on the practice tests until you're ready. If you take a test on your first day of study, you may be overwhelmed by the amount of material covered and how much you need to learn. Work up to it gradually.

On test day, you'll need to be prepared for answering questions, managing your time, and using the test-taking strategies you've learned. It's a lot to balance, like a mental marathon that will have a big impact on your future. Like training for a marathon, you'll need to start slowly and work your way up. When test day arrives, you'll be ready.

Start with the strategies you've read in the first two Secret Keys—plan your course and study in the way that works best for you. If you have time, consider using multiple study resources to get different approaches to the same concepts. It can be helpful to see difficult concepts from more than one angle. Then find a good source for practice tests. Many times, the test website will suggest potential study resources or provide sample tests.

Practice Test Strategy

If you're able to find at least three practice tests, we recommend this strategy:

UNTIMED AND OPEN-BOOK PRACTICE

Take the first test with no time constraints and with your notes and study guide handy. Take your time and focus on applying the strategies you've learned.

TIMED AND OPEN-BOOK PRACTICE

Take the second practice test open-book as well, but set a timer and practice pacing yourself to finish in time.

TIMED AND CLOSED-BOOK PRACTICE

Take any other practice tests as if it were test day. Set a timer and put away your study materials. Sit at a table or desk in a quiet room, imagine yourself at the testing center, and answer questions as quickly and accurately as possible.

Keep repeating timed and closed-book tests on a regular basis until you run out of practice tests or it's time for the actual test. Your mind will be ready for the schedule and stress of test day, and you'll be able to focus on recalling the material you've learned.

Secret Key #4 – Pace Yourself

Once you're fully prepared for the material on the test, your biggest challenge on test day will be managing your time. Just knowing that the clock is ticking can make you panic even if you have plenty of time left. Work on pacing yourself so you can build confidence against the time constraints of the exam. Pacing is a difficult skill to master, especially in a high-pressure environment, so **practice is vital**.

Set time expectations for your pace based on how much time is available. For example, if a section has 60 questions and the time limit is 30 minutes, you know you have to average 30 seconds or less per question in order to answer them all. Although 30 seconds is the hard limit, set 25 seconds per question as your goal, so you reserve extra time to spend on harder questions. When you budget extra time for the harder questions, you no longer have any reason to stress when those questions take longer to answer.

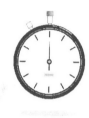

Don't let this time expectation distract you from working through the test at a calm, steady pace, but keep it in mind so you don't spend too much time on any one question. Recognize that taking extra time on one question you don't understand may keep you from answering two that you do understand later in the test. If your time limit for a question is up and you're still not sure of the answer, mark it and move on, and come back to it later if the time and the test format allow. If the testing format doesn't allow you to return to earlier questions, just make an educated guess; then put it out of your mind and move on.

On the easier questions, be careful not to rush. It may seem wise to hurry through them so you have more time for the challenging ones, but it's not worth missing one if you know the concept and just didn't take the time to read the question fully. Work efficiently but make sure you understand the question and have looked at all of the answer choices, since more than one may seem right at first.

Even if you're paying attention to the time, you may find yourself a little behind at some point. You should speed up to get back on track, but do so wisely. Don't panic; just take a few seconds less on each question until you're caught up. Don't guess without thinking, but do look through the answer choices and eliminate any you know are wrong. If you can get down to two choices, it is often worthwhile to guess from those. Once you've chosen an answer, move on and don't dwell on any that you skipped or had to hurry through. If a question was taking too long, chances are it was one of the harder ones, so you weren't as likely to get it right anyway.

On the other hand, if you find yourself getting ahead of schedule, it may be beneficial to slow down a little. The more quickly you work, the more likely you are to make a careless mistake that will affect your score. You've budgeted time for each question, so don't be afraid to spend that time. Practice an efficient but careful pace to get the most out of the time you have.

Secret Key #5 – Have a Plan for Guessing

When you're taking the test, you may find yourself stuck on a question. Some of the answer choices seem better than others, but you don't see the one answer choice that is obviously correct. What do you do?

The scenario described above is very common, yet most test takers have not effectively prepared for it. Developing and practicing a plan for guessing may be one of the single most effective uses of your time as you get ready for the exam.

In developing your plan for guessing, there are three questions to address:

- When should you start the guessing process?
- How should you narrow down the choices?
- Which answer should you choose?

When to Start the Guessing Process

Unless your plan for guessing is to select C every time (which, despite its merits, is not what we recommend), you need to leave yourself enough time to apply your answer elimination strategies. Since you have a limited amount of time for each question, that means that if you're going to give yourself the best shot at guessing correctly, you have to decide quickly whether or not you will guess.

Of course, the best-case scenario is that you don't have to guess at all, so first, see if you can answer the question based on your knowledge of the subject and basic reasoning skills. Focus on the key words in the question and try to jog your memory of related topics. Give yourself a chance to bring the knowledge to mind, but once you realize that you don't have (or you can't access) the knowledge you need to answer the question, it's time to start the guessing process.

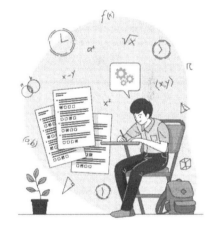

It's almost always better to start the guessing process too early than too late. It only takes a few seconds to remember something and answer the question from knowledge. Carefully eliminating wrong answer choices takes longer. Plus, going through the process of eliminating answer choices can actually help jog your memory.

Summary: Start the guessing process as soon as you decide that you can't answer the question based on your knowledge.

7

How to Narrow Down the Choices

The next chapter in this book (**Test-Taking Strategies**) includes a wide range of strategies for how to approach questions and how to look for answer choices to eliminate. You will definitely want to read those carefully, practice them, and figure out which ones work best for you. Here though, we're going to address a mindset rather than a particular strategy.

Your odds of guessing an answer correctly depend on how many options you are choosing from.

Number of options left	5	4	3	2	1
Odds of guessing correctly	20%	25%	33%	50%	100%

You can see from this chart just how valuable it is to be able to eliminate incorrect answers and make an educated guess, but there are two things that many test takers do that cause them to miss out on the benefits of guessing:

- Accidentally eliminating the correct answer
- Selecting an answer based on an impression

We'll look at the first one here, and the second one in the next section.

To avoid accidentally eliminating the correct answer, we recommend a thought exercise called **the $5 challenge**. In this challenge, you only eliminate an answer choice from contention if you are willing to bet $5 on it being wrong. Why $5? Five dollars is a small but not insignificant amount of money. It's an amount you could afford to lose but wouldn't want to throw away. And while losing $5 once might not

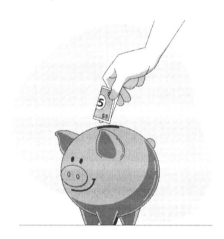

hurt too much, doing it twenty times will set you back $100. In the same way, each small decision you make—eliminating a choice here, guessing on a question there—won't by itself impact your score very much, but when you put them all together, they can make a big difference. By holding each answer choice elimination decision to a higher standard, you can reduce the risk of accidentally eliminating the correct answer.

The $5 challenge can also be applied in a positive sense: If you are willing to bet $5 that an answer choice *is* correct, go ahead and mark it as correct.

Summary: Only eliminate an answer choice if you are willing to bet $5 that it is wrong.

Which Answer to Choose

You're taking the test. You've run into a hard question and decided you'll have to guess. You've eliminated all the answer choices you're willing to bet $5 on. Now you have to pick an answer. Why do we even need to talk about this? Why can't you just pick whichever one you feel like when the time comes?

The answer to these questions is that if you don't come into the test with a plan, you'll rely on your impression to select an answer choice, and if you do that, you risk falling into a trap. The test writers know that everyone who takes their test will be guessing on some of the questions, so they intentionally write wrong answer choices to seem plausible. You still have to pick an answer though, and if the wrong answer choices are designed to look right, how can you ever be sure that you're not falling for their trap? The best solution we've found to this dilemma is to take the decision out of your hands entirely. Here is the process we recommend:

Once you've eliminated any choices that you are confident (willing to bet $5) are wrong, select the first remaining choice as your answer.

Whether you choose to select the first remaining choice, the second, or the last, the important thing is that you use some preselected standard. Using this approach guarantees that you will not be enticed into selecting an answer choice that looks right, because you are not basing your decision on how the answer choices look.

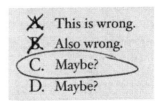

This is not meant to make you question your knowledge. Instead, it is to help you recognize the difference between your knowledge and your impressions. There's a huge difference between thinking an answer is right because of what you know, and thinking an answer is right because it looks or sounds like it should be right.

Summary: To ensure that your selection is appropriately random, make a predetermined selection from among all answer choices you have not eliminated.

Test-Taking Strategies

This section contains a list of test-taking strategies that you may find helpful as you work through the test. By taking what you know and applying logical thought, you can maximize your chances of answering any question correctly!

It is very important to realize that every question is different and every person is different: no single strategy will work on every question, and no single strategy will work for every person. That's why we've included all of them here, so you can try them out and determine which ones work best for different types of questions and which ones work best for you.

Question Strategies

⊘ READ CAREFULLY

Read the question and the answer choices carefully. Don't miss the question because you misread the terms. You have plenty of time to read each question thoroughly and make sure you understand what is being asked. Yet a happy medium must be attained, so don't waste too much time. You must read carefully and efficiently.

⊘ CONTEXTUAL CLUES

Look for contextual clues. If the question includes a word you are not familiar with, look at the immediate context for some indication of what the word might mean. Contextual clues can often give you all the information you need to decipher the meaning of an unfamiliar word. Even if you can't determine the meaning, you may be able to narrow down the possibilities enough to make a solid guess at the answer to the question.

⊘ PREFIXES

If you're having trouble with a word in the question or answer choices, try dissecting it. Take advantage of every clue that the word might include. Prefixes can be a huge help. Usually, they allow you to determine a basic meaning. *Pre-* means before, *post-* means after, *pro-* is positive, *de-* is negative. From prefixes, you can get an idea of the general meaning of the word and try to put it into context.

⊘ HEDGE WORDS

Watch out for critical hedge words, such as *likely, may, can, sometimes, often, almost, mostly, usually, generally, rarely,* and *sometimes.* Question writers insert these hedge phrases to cover every possibility. Often an answer choice will be wrong simply because it leaves no room for exception. Be on guard for answer choices that have definitive words such as *exactly* and *always.*

⊘ SWITCHBACK WORDS

Stay alert for *switchbacks.* These are the words and phrases frequently used to alert you to shifts in thought. The most common switchback words are *but, although,* and *however.* Others include *nevertheless, on the other hand, even though, while, in spite of, despite,* and *regardless of.* Switchback words are important to catch because they can change the direction of the question or an answer choice.

⊘ FACE VALUE

When in doubt, use common sense. Accept the situation in the problem at face value. Don't read too much into it. These problems will not require you to make wild assumptions. If you have to go beyond creativity and warp time or space in order to have an answer choice fit the question, then you should move on and

10

consider the other answer choices. These are normal problems rooted in reality. The applicable relationship or explanation may not be readily apparent, but it is there for you to figure out. Use your common sense to interpret anything that isn't clear.

Answer Choice Strategies

⊘ ANSWER SELECTION

The most thorough way to pick an answer choice is to identify and eliminate wrong answers until only one is left, then confirm it is the correct answer. Sometimes an answer choice may immediately seem right, but be careful. The test writers will usually put more than one reasonable answer choice on each question, so take a second to read all of them and make sure that the other choices are not equally obvious. As long as you have time left, it is better to read every answer choice than to pick the first one that looks right without checking the others.

⊘ ANSWER CHOICE FAMILIES

An answer choice family consists of two (in rare cases, three) answer choices that are very similar in construction and cannot all be true at the same time. If you see two answer choices that are direct opposites or parallels, one of them is usually the correct answer. For instance, if one answer choice says that quantity x increases and another either says that quantity x decreases (opposite) or says that quantity y increases (parallel), then those answer choices would fall into the same family. An answer choice that doesn't match the construction of the answer choice family is more likely to be incorrect. Most questions will not have answer choice families, but when they do appear, you should be prepared to recognize them.

⊘ ELIMINATE ANSWERS

Eliminate answer choices as soon as you realize they are wrong, but make sure you consider all possibilities. If you are eliminating answer choices and realize that the last one you are left with is also wrong, don't panic. Start over and consider each choice again. There may be something you missed the first time that you will realize on the second pass.

⊘ AVOID FACT TRAPS

Don't be distracted by an answer choice that is factually true but doesn't answer the question. You are looking for the choice that answers the question. Stay focused on what the question is asking for so you don't accidentally pick an answer that is true but incorrect. Always go back to the question and make sure the answer choice you've selected actually answers the question and is not merely a true statement.

⊘ EXTREME STATEMENTS

In general, you should avoid answers that put forth extreme actions as standard practice or proclaim controversial ideas as established fact. An answer choice that states the "process should be used in certain situations, if..." is much more likely to be correct than one that states the "process should be discontinued completely." The first is a calm rational statement and doesn't even make a definitive, uncompromising stance, using a hedge word *if* to provide wiggle room, whereas the second choice is far more extreme.

⊘ BENCHMARK

As you read through the answer choices and you come across one that seems to answer the question well, mentally select that answer choice. This is not your final answer, but it's the one that will help you evaluate the other answer choices. The one that you selected is your benchmark or standard for judging each of the other answer choices. Every other answer choice must be compared to your benchmark. That choice is correct until proven otherwise by another answer choice beating it. If you find a better answer,

11

then that one becomes your new benchmark. Once you've decided that no other choice answers the question as well as your benchmark, you have your final answer.

⊘ PREDICT THE ANSWER

Before you even start looking at the answer choices, it is often best to try to predict the answer. When you come up with the answer on your own, it is easier to avoid distractions and traps because you will know exactly what to look for. The right answer choice is unlikely to be word-for-word what you came up with, but it should be a close match. Even if you are confident that you have the right answer, you should still take the time to read each option before moving on.

General Strategies

⊘ TOUGH QUESTIONS

If you are stumped on a problem or it appears too hard or too difficult, don't waste time. Move on! Remember though, if you can quickly check for obviously incorrect answer choices, your chances of guessing correctly are greatly improved. Before you completely give up, at least try to knock out a couple of possible answers. Eliminate what you can and then guess at the remaining answer choices before moving on.

⊘ CHECK YOUR WORK

Since you will probably not know every term listed and the answer to every question, it is important that you get credit for the ones that you do know. Don't miss any questions through careless mistakes. If at all possible, try to take a second to look back over your answer selection and make sure you've selected the correct answer choice and haven't made a costly careless mistake (such as marking an answer choice that you didn't mean to mark). This quick double check should more than pay for itself in caught mistakes for the time it costs.

⊘ PACE YOURSELF

It's easy to be overwhelmed when you're looking at a page full of questions; your mind is confused and full of random thoughts, and the clock is ticking down faster than you would like. Calm down and maintain the pace that you have set for yourself. Especially as you get down to the last few minutes of the test, don't let the small numbers on the clock make you panic. As long as you are on track by monitoring your pace, you are guaranteed to have time for each question.

⊘ DON'T RUSH

It is very easy to make errors when you are in a hurry. Maintaining a fast pace in answering questions is pointless if it makes you miss questions that you would have gotten right otherwise. Test writers like to include distracting information and wrong answers that seem right. Taking a little extra time to avoid careless mistakes can make all the difference in your test score. Find a pace that allows you to be confident in the answers that you select.

⊘ KEEP MOVING

Panicking will not help you pass the test, so do your best to stay calm and keep moving. Taking deep breaths and going through the answer elimination steps you practiced can help to break through a stress barrier and keep your pace.

Final Notes

The combination of a solid foundation of content knowledge and the confidence that comes from practicing your plan for applying that knowledge is the key to maximizing your performance on test day. As your foundation of content knowledge is built up and strengthened, you'll find that the strategies included in this chapter become more and more effective in helping you quickly sift through the distractions and traps of the test to isolate the correct answer.

Now that you're preparing to move forward into the test content chapters of this book, be sure to keep your goal in mind. As you read, think about how you will be able to apply this information on the test. If you've already seen sample questions for the test and you have an idea of the question format and style, try to come up with questions of your own that you can answer based on what you're reading. This will give you valuable practice applying your knowledge in the same ways you can expect to on test day.

Good luck and good studying!

Clinical Practice

Head and Neck

TBI

Traumatic brain injury (TBI) occurs when an external force damages the brain, thereby causing an alteration in its function. TBIs can be classified as mild, moderate or severe. Common causes of traumatic brain injury include falls, motor vehicle accidents, and assaults. Traumatic brain injuries are more common in males than females.

- **Signs and symptoms**: Signs and symptoms of a traumatic brain injury may not be immediately present, depending on the severity of the injury. Symptoms may be subtle initially and then worsen. Symptoms include: loss of consciousness, headache, blurred vision, confusion, nausea, vomiting, fatigue, somnolence, dizziness, loss of balance or coordination, seizures, tinnitus, slurred speech and photosensitivity.
- **Diagnosis**: X-rays of the spine, CT and MRI of the head, and angiography if penetrating injury occurred. The Glasgow coma scale is most commonly used to assess neurologic status in the TBI patient.
- **Treatment**: Treatment of TBI includes frequent monitoring of vital signs, fluid balance and neurologic status. Intracranial pressure may also be monitored. Mannitol and hypertonic saline may be administered to decrease intracranial pressure and cerebral edema. Antiepileptic medications may be utilized to prevent or minimize seizure activity. In cases of severe injury, decompressive craniotomy and initiation of a hypothermia protocol may be used to reduce intracranial pressure, cerebral edema and cell death.

BLUNT HEAD TRAUMA

Head trauma can occur as the result from intentional or unintentional blunt or penetrating trauma, such as from falls, automobile accidents, sports injuries, or violence. The degree of injury correlates with the impact force. The skull provides protection to the brain, but a severe blow can cause significant neurological damage. Blunt trauma can include:

- **Acceleration-deceleration injuries** are those in which a blow to the stationary head causes the elastic skull to change shape, pushing against the brain, which moves sharply backward in response, striking against the skull.
- **Bruising** can occur at the point of impact (*coup*) and the point where the brain hits the skull (*contrecoup*). So a blow to the frontal area can cause damage to the occipital region.

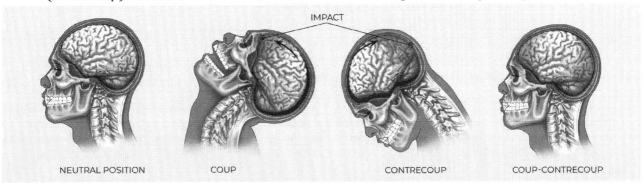

IMPACT

NEUTRAL POSITION   COUP   CONTRECOUP   COUP-CONTRECOUP

15

- **Shear injuries,** where vessels are torn, results from sudden movement of the brain.
- **Severe compression** may force the brain through the tentorial opening, damaging the brainstem.

COMPLICATIONS OF HEAD TRAUMA
FRACTURES

Fractures are a common cause of penetrating wounds causing cerebral lacerations. Open fractures are those in which the dura is torn, and closed is when the dura remain intact. While fractures by themselves do not cause neurological damage, force is needed to fracture the skull, often causing damage to underlying structures. Meningeal arteries lie in grooves on the underside of the skull, and a fracture can cause an arterial tear and hemorrhage. Skull fractures include:

- **Basilar**: Occurs in bones at the base of the brain and can cause severe brainstem damage. May see bruising around the ear ("Battles sign") and leaking of CSF from nose and ears (bloody fluid will develop a ring of clear fluid when placed on guaze of linens – "Halo sign").
- **Comminuted**: Skull fractures into small pieces.
- **Compound**: Surface laceration extends to include a skull fracture.
- **Depressed**: Pieces of the skull are depressed inward on the brain tissue, often producing dural tears.
- **Linear/hairline:** Skull fracture forms a thin line without any splintering.

CEREBRAL EDEMA AND INCREASED ICP

Head injuries that occur at the time of trauma include **fractures, contusions, hematomas, and diffuse cerebral and vascular injury**. These injuries may result in hypoxia, increased intracranial pressure, and cerebral edema. Open injuries may result in infection. Patients often suffer initial hypertension, which increases intracranial pressure, decreasing perfusion. Often the primary problem with head trauma is a significant increase in swelling, which also interferes with perfusion, causing hypoxia and hypercapnia, which trigger increased blood flow. This increased volume at a time when injury impairs auto-regulation increases cerebral edema, which, in turn, increases intracranial pressure and results in a further decrease in perfusion with resultant ischemia. If pressure continues to rise, the brain may herniate. Concomitant hypotension may result in hypoventilation, further complicating treatment. Treatments include:

- Monitoring ICP and CCP.
- Providing oxygen.
- Elevating the head of the bed and maintaining proper body alignment.
- Giving medications: Analgesics, anticonvulsants, and anesthetics.
- Providing blood/fluids to stabilize hemodynamics.
- Managing airway, providing mechanical ventilation if needed.
- Providing osmotic agents, such as mannitol and hypertonic saline solution, to reduce cerebral edema.

CONCUSSIONS, CONTUSIONS, AND LACERATIONS
A variety of different injuries can occur as a result of **head trauma**:

- **Concussions** are diffuse areas of bleeding in the brain, one of the most common injuries and are usually relatively transient, causing no permanent neurological damage. They may result in confusion, disorientation, and mild amnesia, which last only minutes or hours.

- **Contusions/lacerations** are bruising and tears of cerebral tissue. There may be petechial areas at the impact site (coup) or larger bruising. Contrecoup injuries are less common in children than in adults. Areas most impacted by contusions and lacerations are the occipital, frontal, and temporal lobes. The degree of injury relates to the amount of vascular damage, but initial symptoms are similar to concussion; however, symptoms persist and may progress, depending upon the degree of injury. Lacerations are often caused by fractures.

PENETRATING HEAD TRAUMA

Penetrating head trauma most often results from gunshot wounds, stab wounds (knife, scissors, spikes), motor-vehicle accidents, and work-related accidents (such as nail gun or screwdriver injuries). Penetrating head trauma may result in skull fractures and traumatic brain injury through lacerations in the parenchyma, compression of tissue, cavitation, and secondary trauma. With penetrating injury, there is a breach in the cranium with the possibility of the projectile remaining. If the projectile exits, the wound is classified as a perforation. Perforating wounds tend to be more severe than penetrating because perforating wounds result in permanent cavitation as some tissue is expelled with the projectile. The location and degree of penetrating injuries may vary widely. Stab wounds tend to result in more localized injury (slot wounds), and survival rates are better if the instrument of injury is in place rather than removed before treatment. Treatment varies widely and includes observation, antibiotics, surgical repair, and treatment to relieve pressure and reduce intracranial pressure.

HEMORRHAGIC STROKES

Hemorrhagic strokes account for about 20% of all strokes and result from a ruptured cerebral artery, causing not only lack of oxygen and nutrients but also edema that causes widespread pressure and damage:

- **Intracerebral** is bleeding into the substance of the brain from an artery in the central lobes, basal ganglia, pons, or cerebellum. Intracerebral hemorrhage usually results from atherosclerotic degenerative changes, hypertension, brain tumors, anticoagulation therapy, or use of illicit drugs, such as cocaine.
- **Intracranial aneurysm** occurs with ballooning cerebral artery ruptures, most commonly at the Circle of Willis.
- **Arteriovenous malformation**. Rupture of AVMs is a cause of brain attack in young adults.
- **Subarachnoid hemorrhage** is bleeding in the space between the meninges and brain, resulting from aneurysm, AVM, or trauma. This type of hemorrhage compresses brain tissue.

TREATMENT

The patient may need airway protection/artificial ventilation if neurologic compromise is severe. Blood pressure is lowered to control rate of bleeding, but with caution to avoid hypotension and resulting cerebral ischemia (Goal – CPP >70). Sedation can lower ICP and blood pressure, and seizure prophylaxis will be indicated as blood irritates the cerebral cells. An intraventricular catheter may be used in ICP management; correct any clotting disorders if identified.

INTRACRANIAL/INTRAVENTRICULAR HEMORRHAGE

EPIDURAL AND SUBDURAL

Epidural hemorrhage is bleeding between the dura and the skull, pushing the brain downward and inward. The hemorrhage is usually caused by arterial tears, so bleeding is often rapid, leading to severe neurological deficits and respiratory arrest.

Subdural hemorrhage is bleeding between the dura and the cerebrum, usually from tears in the cortical veins of the subdural space. It tends to develop more slowly than epidural hemorrhage and can result in a subdural hematoma. If the bleeding is acute and develops within minutes or hours of injury, the prognosis is poor. Subacute hematomas that develop more slowly cause varying degrees of injury. Subdural hemorrhage is a common injury related to trauma but it can result from coagulopathies or aneurysms. Symptoms of acute injury may occur within 24-48 hours, but subacute bleeding may not be evident for up to 2 weeks after injury. Chronic hemorrhage occurs primarily in the elderly. Symptoms vary and may include bradycardia, tachycardia, hypertension, and alterations in consciousness. Older children and adults usually require surgical evacuation of the hematoma.

SUBARACHNOID

Subarachnoid hemorrhage (SAH) may occur after trauma but is common from rupture of a berry aneurysm or an arteriovenous malformation (AVM). However, there are a number of disorders that may be implicated: neoplasms, sickle cell disease, infection, hemophilia, and leukemia. The first presenting symptom may be complaints of severe headache, nausea and vomiting, nuchal rigidity, palsy related to cranial nerve compression, retinal hemorrhages, and papilledema. Late complications include hyponatremia and hydrocephalus. Symptoms worsen as intracranial pressure rises. SAH from aneurysm is classified as follows:

- **Grade I:** No symptoms or slight headache and nuchal rigidity.
- **Grade II:** Mod-severe headache with nuchal rigidity and cranial nerve palsy.
- **Grade III:** Drowsy, progressing to confusion or mild focal deficits.
- **Grade IV**: Stupor, with hemiparesis (mod-severe), early decerebrate rigidity, and vegetative disturbances.
- **Grade V:** Coma state with decerebrate rigidity.

Treatment includes:

- Identifying and treating underlying cause.
- Observing for re-bleeding.
- Anti-seizure medications (such as levetiracetam or phenytoin) to control seizures.
- Antihypertensives.
- Surgical repair if indicated.

CEREBRAL HYPOXIA

Cerebral hypoxia (hypoxic encephalopathy) occurs when the oxygen supply to the brain is decreased. If hypoxia is mild, the brain compensates by increasing cerebral blood flow, but it can only double in volume and cannot compensate for severe hypoxic conditions. Hypoxia may be the result of insufficient oxygen in the environment, inadequate exchange at the alveolar level of the lungs, or inadequate circulation to the brain. Brain cells may begin dying within 5 minutes if deprived of adequate oxygenation, so any condition or trauma that interferes with oxygenation can result in brain damage:

- Near-drowning.
- Asphyxia.
- Cardiac arrest.
- High altitude sickness.
- Carbon monoxide.
- Diseases that interfere with respiration, such as myasthenia gravis and amyotrophic lateral sclerosis.
- Anesthesia complications.

Symptoms include increasing neurological deficits, depending upon the degree and area of damage, with changes in mentation that range from confusion to coma. Prompt identification of the cause and increase in perfusion to the brain is critical for survival.

CEREBRAL ANEURYSMS

Cerebral aneurysms, weakening and dilation of a cerebral artery, are usually congenital (90%) while the remaining (10%) result from direct trauma or infection. Aneurysms usually range from 2-7 mm and occur in the Circle of Willis at the base of the brain. A rupturing aneurysm may decrease perfusion as well as increasing pressure on surrounding brain tissue. Cerebral aneurysms are classified as follows:

- **Berry/saccular:** The most common congenital type occurs at a bifurcation and grows from the base on a stem, usually at the Circle of Willis.
- **Fusiform**: Large and irregular (>2.5 cm) and rarely ruptures but causes increased intracranial pressure. Usually involves the internal carotid or vertebrobasilar artery.
- **Mycotic**: Rare type that occurs secondary to bacterial infection and aseptic emboli.
- **Dissecting**: Wall is torn apart and blood enters layers. This may occur during angiography or secondary to trauma or disease.
- **Traumatic Charcot-Bouchard (pseudoaneurysm):** small lesion resulting from chronic hypertension.

BRAIN DEATH

While each state has its own laws that describe the legal definition of **brain death,** most include some variation of this description:

- Brain death has occurred if the person has "sustained irreversible cessation of circulatory and respiratory functions; or has sustained irreversible cessation of all functions of the entire brain, including the brain stem."

Some states specify the number of physicians that must make the determination and others simply say the decision must be made in accordance with accepted medical practice. Criteria for determination of brain death include coma or lack of responsiveness, apnea (without ventilation), and absence of brainstem reflexes. In many states, findings must be confirmed by at least 2 physicians. **Tests used to confirm brain death** include:

- Cerebral angiograms: Delayed intracerebral filling or obstruction.
- EEG: Lack of response to auditory, visual, or somatic stimuli.
- Ultrasound (transcranial): Abnormal/lack of flow.
- Cerebral scintograms: Static images at preset time intervals.
- Absence of oculoscephalic reflex ("Doll's eyes"): patients eyes stay fixed when head is turned side to side
- Absence of oculovestibular Reflex ("cold caloric"): When ice cold water is injected into the ear, the patient's eyes exhibit no response. The patient's HOB must be atleast 20° for this test to be accurate.

SPINAL CORD INJURIES

Spinal cord injuries may result from blunt trauma (such as automobile accidents), falls from a height, sports injuries, and penetrating trauma (such as gunshot or knife wounds). Damage results from mechanical injury and secondary responses resulting from hemorrhage, edema, and ischemia. The type of symptoms relates to the area and degree of injury. About 50% of spinal cord injuries involve the cervical spine between C4 and C7 with a 20% mortality rate, and 50% of injuries result in quadriplegia.

Neurogenic shock may occur with injury above T6, with bradycardia, hypotension, and autonomic instability. Patients may develop hypoxia because of respiratory dysfunction. With high injuries, up to 70% of patients will require a tracheostomy (especially at or above C3). Patients with paralysis are at high risk for pressure sores, urinary tract infections (from catheterization), and constipation/impaction.

TYPES

Types of spinal cord injuries include:

- **Complete transection**: Paralysis (hemiplegia, quadriplegia) below the area of transection with complete lack of sensation and motor control. Injury at T6 or above, results in spinal shock with flaccid paralysis below lesion with loss of sensations and rectal and bladder tone, bradycardia, and hypotension. Prognosis is poor.
- **Anterior cord**: The posterior column functions remain, so there is sensation of touch, vibration, and position remaining below injury but with complete paralysis and loss of sensations of pain and temperature. Prognosis is poor.
- **Brown-Séguard**: The cord is hemisected resulting in spastic paresis, loss of sense of position and vibration on the injured side and loss of pain and temperature on the other side. Prognosis is good.
- **Cauda equina**: Damage is below L-1 with variable loss of motor ability and sensation, and bowel and bladder dysfunction. Injury is to peripheral nerves, which can regenerate so prognosis is better than for other lesions of the spinal cord.
- **Central cord**: Results from hyperextension and ischemia or stenosis of the cervical spine, causing quadriparesis (more severe in upper extremities) with some loss of sensations of pain and temperature. Prognosis is good but fine motor skills are often impaired in upper extremities.
- **Conus medullaris**: Injury to lower spine (lower lumbar and sacral nerves).
- **Posterior cord**: Motor function is preserved but without sensation.

JAW FRACTURES

The bones of the jaw include the maxilla (which is fixed) and the mandible (which is moveable), and both generally contain teeth. Jaw injuries are most often caused by blunt trauma, such as in motor vehicle accidents, falls from height, or assault:

- **Maxillary injuries:** Typical maxillary injury includes dentoalveolar trauma with dislodged, missing, or impacted teeth. Intraoral radiographs or CT scans are used to assess injury, as other injuries are common. Treatment may be conservative with antibiotics and observation, but if the patient has vision impairment, numbness, change in appearance, or other complications, surgical repair with fixation may be necessary.
- **Mandibular injuries**: Mandibular fractures may result in airway obstruction (requiring emergent intervention), swelling, bleeding, and paresthesia of lip and chin. Treatment depends on the location and extent of the fracture and may involve resting the mandible by avoiding solid or hard-to-chew foods or more extensive surgical repair that involves placing metal plates about the fracture or wiring the jaws together to prevent movement, necessitating a liquid diet.

BLUNT OCULAR TRAUMA

Blunt ocular trauma occurs with impact to the eye that may occur with motor vehicle accidents, sports accidents, work-related injuries (especially construction), and assaults (fist impact). Following impact, signs and symptoms may include swelling, redness, bruising about the eye, pain, blurred vision, loss of vision, photophobia, floaters, flashes, and tearing. Blunt trauma can result in rupture of the sclera and corneal abrasions. Orbital blowout fractures or other head injuries may also be present. Diagnosis of the type and degree of injury may include CT scan, ophthalmoscopy, and/or ultrasound. Treatment depends on the injury. Options include:

- **Corneal abrasions**: Ophthalmic antibiotic ointment.
- **Traumatic optic neuropathy** (may result in complete blindness): Steroids are generally now avoided as they may increase risk of mortality in patients with brain injury, and studies have not supported their efficacy. Surgical decompression may be considered but has potential risks and is not always effective.
- **Globe rupture**: Protect eye and prepare for emergent surgical repair.
- Retinal detachment: Surgical repair.
- **Hyphema:** Usually resolves within 7 days. Mydriatics for comfort, topical beta-blockers for increased intraocular pressure.

PENETRATING OCULAR TRAUMA

Penetrating ocular trauma may be obvious on examination, especially if involving gunshot or knife injuries, which are generally emergent situations that require surgical repair and may involve multiple other injuries. However, other types of penetrating ocular traumas may result from work injuries (usually involving projectiles), contact with a sharp object (such as a thorn, needle, or toy), or a foreign body in the eye. Symptoms may include loss of visual acuity, pain, tearing, blepharospasm, and photophobia. Injuries include:

- **Lacerations**: May be conjunctival, corneoscleral, or eyelid: Conjunctival lacerations >1 cm may need suturing. Corneoscleral repair is usually done in surgery, and eyelid lacerations are sutured.
- **Perforations**: May be single or multiple, and treatment depends on severity of injuries, but usually includes antibiotic ophthalmic ointment. Surgical repair may be necessary
- **Corneal foreign bodies** (usually glass or metal). May lodge in surface of cornea, resulting in pain and tearing. The foreign body is removed with a 21G needle after instillation of topical anesthetic under slit-lamp magnification, followed by eye patching and ophthalmic antibiotic ointment to prevent infection. Deep foreign bodies require surgical removal

PENETRATING LARYNGEAL TRAUMA

Penetrating laryngeal trauma most often results from stab or gunshot wounds or blast injuries and is associated with penetrating neck trauma. The extent of injury may vary from very mild to life-threatening. Indications of laryngeal trauma includes painful or difficulty swallowing, hoarseness, pain, dyspnea, stridor, tracheal deviation, bruising, hemoptysis, bleeding, obvious wound, and absent laryngeal crepitus. Injury related to knife wounds is usually restricted to the path of the blade; however, gunshot wounds may cause severe destruction of tissue, including damage to the neck and major vessels in the neck. If active bleeding is present, direct pressure should be applied and fluid resuscitation carried out to stabilize the patient for surgical repair, which is commonly necessary for penetrating wounds unless very minor. Diagnostic procedures include radiographs to rule out other injuries (such as injuries of the cervical vertebrae/spine) or complications, CT scan, and flexible fiberoptic laryngoscopy. Patients are generally treated with antibiotics and may require tracheotomy and/or stenting.

Trunk

PENETRATING CARDIAC INJURIES

The incidence of **penetrating cardiac injuries** has been on the rise, primarily associated with gun shot injuries and stabbings. The extent of damage caused by a stab wound is often easier to assess than gunshot wounds, which may be multiple and often results in unpredictable and widespread damage not only to the heart but other structures. Mortality rates are very high in the first hour after a penetrating cardiac injury, so it is imperative that the patient be taken immediately to a trauma center rather than attempts made to stabilize the person at the site. NEVER attempt to remove the object in the field/without a physican present. The **primary complications**:

- **Exsanguination** is frequently related to gunshot wounds, and prognosis is very poor. This may lead to hemothorax and hemorrhagic shock.
- **Cardiac tamponade** is more common with knife wounds, but prognosis is fairly good with surgical repair. Cardiac tamponade often presents with three classic symptoms, known as Beck's triad that should be quickly recognized: muffled heart sounds, low arterial blood pressure, and jugular vein distention.
- **Pneumothorax**: deviated trachea, increasing SVR, tachypnea and anxiety all may indicate tension pneumothorax, which is a medical emergency. It is treated by emergent insertion of chest tube or needle aspiration of trapped air. Open wounds can be emergently dressed with a three-sided dressing until chest tube can be inserted to create a "flutter valve" effect and allow trapped air to escape.

Nursing Considerations: Management includes controlling bleeding, giving fluids and pressors for blood pressure, preparing patient for surgery, and monitoring for the above mentioned complications.

BLUNT CARDIAC INJURIES

Blunt cardiac trauma most often occurs as the result of motor vehicle accidents, falls, or other blows to the chest, which can result in respiratory distress as well as hypovolemia from rupture of the great vessels of the heart and/or cardiac failure from cardiac tamponade or increasing intrathoracic pressure. The heart is particularly vulnerable to chest trauma, with the right atrium and right ventricle the most commonly injured because they are anterior to the rest of the heart. Cardiac trauma may be difficult to diagnose because of other injuries, but if suspected, an ECG should be done and if any abnormalities (dysrhythmias, ST changes, sinus tachycardia, or heart block) are present, continuous monitoring should be utilized for 24-48 hours. An echocardiogram may be done to evaluate cardiac function. Decreased cardiac output and cerebral oxygenation may result in severe agitation with combative behavior, so changes in mentation should be monitored. Medications may be needed to control arrhythmias.

ACUTE CORONARY SYNDROMES

Acute coronary syndrome (ACS) is the impairment of blood flow through the coronary arteries, leading to ischemia of the cardiac muscle.

ANGINA

Angina frequently occurs in ACS, manifesting as crushing pain substernally, radiating down the left arm or both arms. However, in females, elderly, and diabetics, symptoms may appear less acute and include nausea, shortness of breath, fatigue, pain/weakness/numbness in arms, or no pain at all (*silent ischemia*). There are multiple **classifications of angina:**

- **Stable angina:** exercise-induced, short lived, relieved by rest or nitroglycerin. Other precipitating events include decrease in environmental temperature, heavy eating, strong emotions (such as fright or anger), or exertion, including coitus.
- **Unstable angina** (preinfarction or crescendo angina): a change in the pattern of stable angina, characterized by an increase in pain, not responding to a single nitroglycerin or rest, and persisting for >5 minutes. May cause a change in EKG, or indicate rupture of an atherosclerotic plaque/beginning of thrombus formation. Treat as a medical emergency, indicates impending MI.

- **Variant angina** (Prinzmetal's angina): results from spasms of the coronary arteries. Associated with or without atherosclerotic plaques, and is often related to smoking, alcohol, or illicit stimulants, but can occur cyclically and at rest. Elevation of ST segments usually occurs with variant angina. Treatment is nitroglycerin or calcium channel blockers.

Q-WAVE AND NON-Q-WAVE MYOCARDIAL INFARCTIONS

Formerly classified as transmural or non-transmural, myocardial infarctions are now classified as Q-wave or non-Q-wave:

- Q-Wave:
- Characterized by series of abnormal Q waves (wider and deeper) on ECG, especially in the early AM (related to adrenergic activity).
- Infarction is usually prolonged and results in necrosis.
- Coronary occlusion is complete in 80-90%.
- Q-wave MI is often, but not always, transmural.
- Peak CK levels occur in about 27 hours.
- Non-Q-Wave
- Characterized by changes in ST-T wave with ST depression (usually reversible within a few days).
- Usually reperfusion occurs spontaneously, so infarct size is smaller. Contraction necrosis related to reperfusion is common.
- Non-Q-wave MI is usually non-transmural.
- Coronary occlusion is complete in only 20-30%.
- Peak CK levels occur in 12-13 hours.
- Reinfarction is common.

MYOCARDIAL INFARCTIONS

Myocardial infarctions are also classified according to their location and the extent of injury. Transmural myocardial infarction involves the full thickness of the heart muscle, often producing a series of Q waves on ECG. While an MI most frequently damages the left ventricle and the septum, the right ventricle may be damaged as well, depending upon the area of the occlusion:

- **Anterior** (V_2 to V_4): occlusion in the proximal left anterior descending (LAD) or left coronary artery. Reciprocal changes found in leads II, III, aV_F.
- **Lateral** (I, aV_L, V_5, V_6): occlusion of the circumflex coronary artery or branch of left coronary artery. Often causes damage to anterior wall as well; Reciprocal changes found in leads II, III, aV_F.
- **Inferior / diaphragmatic** (II, III, aV_F): occlusion of the right coronary artery and causes conduction malfunctions. Reciprocal changes found in leads I and aV_L.
- **Right ventricular** (V_{4R}, V_{5R}, V_{6R}) occlusion of the proximal section of the right coronary artery and damages the right ventricle and the inferior wall. No reciprocal changes should be noted on an ECG.
- **Posterior** (V_8, V_9): occlusion in the right coronary artery or circumflex artery and may be difficult to diagnose. Reciprocal changes found in V_1-V_4.

CLINICAL MANIFESTATIONS AND DIAGNOSIS

A **myocardial infarction** (commonly known as a "heart attack") occurs when either an embolus or vasospasm blocks blood flow through the coronary arteries, causing tissue ischemia and eventual necrosis. **Clinical manifestations** of myocardial infarction may vary considerably (see *Acute Coronary Syndromes/Angina*). More than half of all patients present with acute MIs with no prior history of cardiovascular disease.

Signs/symptoms: angina with pain in chest that may radiate to neck or arms, palpitations, hypertension or hypotension, dyspnea, pulmonary edema, dependent edema, nausea/vomiting, pallor, skin cold and clammy, diaphoresis, decreased urinary output, neurological/psychological disturbances: anxiety, light-headed, headache, visual abnormalities, slurred speech, and fear.

Diagnosis:

- ECG obtained immediately to monitor heart changes over time. Typical changes include T-wave inversion, elevation of ST segment, abnormal Q waves, tachycardia, bradycardia, and dysrhythmias.
- Echocardiogram: decreased ventricular function possible, especially transmural MI.
- Labs:
  - Troponin: increases within 3-6 hours, peaks 14-20; elevated for up to 1-2 weeks.
  - Creatinine kinase (CK-MB): increases 4-8 hours and peaks at about 24 hours (earlier with thrombolytic therapy or PTCA).
  - Ischemia Modified albumin (IMA): increase within minutes, peak 6 hours and return to baseline; verify with other labs.
  - Myoglobin: increases in 30 minutes-4 hours, peaks 6-7 hours. While an increase is not specific to an MI, a failure to increase can be used to rule out an MI.

PAPILLARY MUSCLE RUPTURE

Papillary muscle rupture is a rare but often deadly complication of myocardial ischemia/infarct. It most commonly occurs with inferior infarcts. The papillary muscles are part of the cardiac wall structure; attached to the lower portion of the ventricles, they are responsible for the opening and closing of the tricuspid and mitral valve and preventing prolapse during systole. Rupture of the papillary muscle can occur with myocardial infarct or ischemia in the area of the heart surrounding the papillary muscle. Since the papillary muscles support the mitral valve, rupture will cause severe mitral regurgitation that may result in cardiogenic shock and subsequent death. Rupture of the papillary muscle may be partial or complete and is considered a life threatening emergency.

- **Signs and symptoms:** Acute heart failure, pulmonary edema and cardiogenic shock - tachycardia, diaphoresis, loss of consciousness, pallor, tachypnea, mental status changes, weak and thready pulse and decreased urinary output.
- **Diagnosis:** Transesophageal echocardiography (TEE) to visualize the papillary muscles, color flow Doppler, echocardiogram and physical assessment. In patients with papillary muscle rupture, a holosystolic murmur starting at the apex and radiating to the axilla may be present.
- **Treatment:** Emergent surgical intervention to repair the mitral valve.

In the cases of complete rupture, patients often experience the rapid development of cardiogenic shock and subsequent death.

ACUTE CARDIAC-RELATED PULMONARY EDEMA

Acute cardiac-related pulmonary edema occurs when heart failure results in fluid overload, leading to third-spacing of fluid into the interstitial spaces of the lungs. Pulmonary edema may result from MI, chronic HF, volume overload, ischemia, or mitral stenosis.

- **Symptoms** include severe dyspnea, cough with blood-tinged frothy sputum, wheezing/rales/crackles on auscultation, cyanosis, and diaphoresis.
- **Diagnosis:** Auscultation, chest x-ray, and echocardiogram.
- **Treatment** includes:

- o Sitting position with 100% oxygen by mask to achieve PO$_2$ >60%.
- o Non-invasive pressure support ventilation (BiPAP) or endotracheal intubation and mechanical ventilation.
- o Morphine sulfate 2-8 mg (IV for severe cases), repeated every 2-4 hours as needed – decreases pre-load and anxiety.
- o IV diuretics (furosemide ≥40 mg or bumetanide ≥1 mg) to provide venous dilation and diuresis.
- o Nitrates as a bolus with an infusion – decrease pre-load.
- o Inhaled β-adrenergic agonists or aminophylline for bronchospasm.
- o Digoxin IV for tachycardia.
- o ACE inhibitors, nitroprusside to reduce afterload.

HYPERTENSIVE CRISES

Hypertensive crises are marked elevations in blood pressure than can cause severe organ damage if left untreated. Hypertensive crises may be caused by endocrine/renal disorders (pheochromocytoma), dissection of an aortic aneurysm, pulmonary edema, subarachnoid hemorrhage, stroke, eclampsia, and medication noncompliance. There are **2 classifications:**

- **Hypertensive emergency** occurs when acute hypertension (1.5 x the 95th percentile), usually >220 systolic and 120 mm Hg diastolic, must be treated immediately to lower blood pressure in order to prevent damage to vital organs.
- **Hypertensive urgency** occurs when acute hypertension must be treated within a few hours but the vital organs are not in immediate danger. Blood pressure is lowered more slowly to avoid hypotension, ischemia of vital organs, or failure of autoregulation. Target is 1/3 reduction over the first 6 hours, 1/3 over next 24 hours, and 1/3 over next 3 days.

Symptoms:

- Basilar HA
- Blurred vision
- Chest pain
- N/V
- SOB
- Seizures
- Ruddy pallor
- Anxiety

Diagnostics:

- ECG
- Chest x-ray
- CBC
- BMP
- Urinalysis (+ blood and casts)

Treatment:

- Medications: vasodilators (Cardene, Nitro, etc.) & diuretics.
- Nursing Interventions: raise HOB to 90°, supplemental O$_2$, frequent neuro checks, teach concerning medication compliance.

ACUTE PERICARDITIS

Pericarditis is inflammation of the pericardial sac with or without increased pericardial fluid. It may be an isolated process or the effect of an underlying disease. If the underlying cause is autoimmune or related to malignancy of some sort, the patient usually presents with symptoms that relate to that disorder. However, most cases are related to a viral etiology, and therefore usually present with flu-like symptoms. Patients that have idiopathic pericarditis or viral pericarditis have a good prognosis with medication alone.

- **Signs/Symptoms:** sharp chest pain, worsened with inspiration and relieved by leaning forward or sitting up (#1- "Mohammad's Sign"), pericardial effusion, respiratory distress, auscultated friction rub, ST elevation/PR depression (progresses to flattened T, inverted T, then return to normal); risk of pericardial effusion
- **Diagnosis:** echocardiogram, ECG, pericardiocentesis or pericardial biopsy, cardiac enzymes (may be mildly elevated), WBC/ESR/CRP all elevated.
- **Treatment:**
  - Medications: NSAIDs for pain / inflammation, Colchicine 0.5 mg twice a day for six months is often prescribed in adjunct to NSAID therapy, as it decreases the incidence of recurrence.
  - Surgery: Pericardiectomy only in extreme cases.

BLUNT CARDIAC TRAUMA AND TRAUMATIC INJURY TO GREAT VESSELS

Blunt cardiac trauma most often occurs as the result of motor vehicle accidents, falls, or other blows to the chest. This can result in respiratory distress, rupture of the great vessels, and cardiac tamponade/increasing intrathoracic pressure. The right atrium and right ventricle are the most commonly injured because they are anterior to the rest of the heart. While not definitive, echocardiogram in conjunction with CPK MB levels is useful in predicting complications. Because diagnosis is challenging until complications appear, every patient with suspected blunt chest trauma should receive an ECG upon admission/STAT. If abnormalities are present, continuous monitoring with should be done for 24-48 hours. Decreased cerebral perfusion/anoxia may result in severe agitation with combative behavior.

Traumatic injuries to the great vessels most commonly result from severe decelerating blunt force or penetrating injuries, with aortic trauma the most common. If the aorta is torn, it will result in almost instant death, but in some cases, there is an incomplete laceration to the intimal lining (innermost membrane) of the aorta, causing an aortic hematoma or bulging. This lining, the adventitia, is quite strong and often will contain the rupture long enough to allow surgical repair.

- **Diagnosis:** chest x-ray or CT; transesophageal echocardiogram to verify.
- **Treatment**: STAT surgical repair to avoid eventual rupture, during which other vessels are examined for clotting or internal injuries.

DISSECTING AORTIC ANEURYSM

A dissecting **aortic aneurysm** occurs when the wall of the aorta is torn and blood flows between the layers of the wall, dilating and weakening it until it risks rupture (which has a 90% mortality). Aortic aneurysms are more than twice as common in males as females, but females have a higher mortality rate, possibly due to increased age at diagnosis. **Abdominal aortic aneurysms (AAA)** are usually related to atherosclerosis, but may also result from Marfan syndrome, Ehlers-Danlos disease, and connective tissue disorders. Rupture usually does not allow time for emergent repair, so identifying and correcting before rupture is essential. Different classification systems are used to describe the type and degree of dissection. Common **classification includes**:

- **DeBakey classification** uses anatomic location as the focal point:
  - *Type I* begins in the ascending aorta but may spread to include the aortic arch and the descending aorta (60%). This is also considered a proximal lesion or Stanford type A.
  - *Type II* is restricted to the ascending aorta (10-15%). This is also considered a proximal lesion or Stanford type A.
  - *Type III* is restricted to the descending aorta (25-30%). This is considered a distal lesion or Stanford type B.

Types I and II are thoracic and type III is abdominal.

AORTIC RUPTURE

Traumatic injuries to the great vessels most commonly result from severe decelerating blunt force or penetrating injuries, with **aortic trauma** the most common. If the aorta is ruptured, it will result in almost instant death, but in some cases, there is an incomplete laceration to the intimal lining (innermost membrane) of the aorta, causing an aortic hematoma or bulging. This lining, the adventitia, is quite strong and often will contain the rupture long enough to allow surgical repair. Thoracic and abdominal aortic aneurysms may also rupture without surgical intervention (surgery indicated when diameter is >5.5 cm to 6 cm). Diagnosis is made initially with chest x-ray or CT, which may show widening of the mediastinum and a misshapen aorta. If there are indications of injury, an aortogram or a combination of CT and transesophageal echocardiogram may be used to verify the injury. Treatment requires surgical repair to avoid eventual rupture, during which other vessels are examined for clotting or internal injuries.

AORTIC ANEURYSMS

Signs/symptoms: often asymptomatic; substernal pain, back pain, dyspnea and/or stridor (from pressure on trachea), cough, distention of neck veins, palpable and pulsating abdominal mass, edema of neck and arms.

Diagnosis: X-ray, CT, MRI, Cardiac cath, TEE/transthoracic echocardiogram,

Treatment:

- **Anti-hypertensives** to reduce systolic BP, such as β-blockers (esmolol) or Alpha-β-blocker combinations (labetalol) to reduce force of blood as it leaves the ventricle to reduce pressure against aortic wall. IV vasodilators (sodium nitroprusside) may also be needed.
- **Intubation and ventilation** may be required if the patient is hemodynamically unstable.
- **Analgesia/sedation** to control anxiety and pain.
- **Surgical repair:** *Type I and II* are usually repaired surgically because of the danger of rupture and cardiac tamponade. *Type III (abdominal)* is often followed medically and surgery only if the aneurysm is >5.5 cm or rapidly expanding. There are two types of surgical repair:
  - **Open:** Patient placed on cardiopulmonary bypass, and through an abdominal incision the damaged portion is removed, and a graft is sutured in place.
  - **Endovascular:** A stent graft is fed through the arteries to line the aorta and exclude the aneurysm.

Complications: myocardial infarction, renal injury, and GI hemorrhage/ischemic bowel, which may occur up to years after surgery. Endo-leaks can occur with a stent graft, increasing risk of rupture.

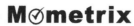

MANAGEMENT OF PULMONARY TRAUMA

PULMONARY HEMORRHAGE

Pulmonary hemorrhage is an acute life-threatening injury that often results in death prior to arrival at the hospital; however, those presenting with traumatic pulmonary hemorrhage, as from a blunt or penetrating injury, requires immediate surgical repair. Even with immediate surgery, survival after serious injury to a major pulmonary vessel is rare. It is important that a large bore IV be immediately inserted and fluid replacement begun while blood is typed and cross matched. The patient should be evaluated for shock and treatment, including colloid solutions, crystalloids, or blood, provided as indicated. Pulmonary hemorrhage may result in hemothorax. In some cases, pneumothorax may also be present, resulting in mediastinal shift that increases the difficulty of identifying and repairing the bleeding vessel. If the patient is stabilized, computed tomography may provide accurate diagnosis to isolate the area of hemorrhage.

TRACHEAL PERFORATION/INJURY

Tracheal perforation/injury may result from external injury, such as from trauma from a vehicle accident or from an assault, such as a gunshot or knife wound or in some cases a laceration as a complication of percutaneous dilation tracheostomy (PDT) or other endotracheal tubes. In some cases, an inhaled foreign object may become lodged in the trachea and eventually erode the tissue. If the injury is severe, respiratory failure may cause death in a very short period of time, so rapid diagnosis and treatment is critical.

Symptoms:

- Severe respiratory distress.
- Hemoptysis.
- Strider with progressive dysphonia.
- Pneumothorax, pneumomediastinum.
- Subcutaneous emphysema from air leaking from the pleural space into the tissues of the chest wall, neck, face, and even into the upper extremities.

Treatment:

- Intubation and non-surgical healing for small lacerations.
- Surgical repair for larger wounds or severe respiratory distress.

PULMONARY CONTUSION

Pulmonary contusion is the result of direct force to the lung, resulting in parenchymal injury and bleeding and edema that impact the capillary-alveoli juncture, resulting in intrapulmonary shunting as the alveoli and interstitium fill with fluid. Parenchymal injury reduces compliance and impairs ventilation. Diagnosis may be more difficult if other injuries, such as fractured ribs or pneumothorax are also present because they may all contribute to respiratory distress. CT scans provide the best diagnostic tool.

Symptoms vary widely depending upon the degree of injury:

- Mild dyspnea/
- Severe progressive dyspnea.
- Hemoptysis.
- Acute respiratory failure.

Treatment varies according to the injury:

- Close monitoring of arterial blood gases and respiratory status.
- Supplemental oxygen.
- Intubation and mechanical ventilation with positive-end expiratory pressure (PEEP) for more severe respiratory distress.
- Fluid management and diuretics to control pulmonary edema.
- Respiratory physiotherapy to clear secretions.

TRAUMATIC ASPHYXIA

Asphyxia may relate to a number of different injuries:

- **Traumatic asphyxia** most commonly involves a crush injury of the thorax, and traumatic injuries to multiple organs may be present. Crush injuries are characterized by petechiae in the area of compression although tight-fitting clothing, such as a woman's bra, may prevent petechiae from forming.
- **Manual strangulation** may involve crush injuries to the throat, such as hyoid fracture. Often the face appears cyanotic while the rest of the body does not. Petechiae may be present on the face as well. Bruising may be noted about the throat.
- **Ligature strangulation** is similar to manual although throat markings are different, with an indented area surrounding the neck.
- **Hanging** produces a V-shaped marking on the throat and does not encircle the neck.
- **Choking** obstructs the airway. (May require bronchoscopy to remove foreign object).

In all cases, immediate establishment of airway, breathing, and circulation (ABCs) takes precedence. Surgical intervention may be needed for traumatic crush injuries.

NEAR-DROWNING ASPHYXIA

Submersion asphyxiation can cause profound damage to the central nervous system, pulmonary dysfunction related to aspiration, cardiac hypoxia with life-threatening arrhythmias, fluid and electrolyte imbalances, and multi-organ damage, so treatment can be complex. Hypothermia related to near drowning has some protective affect because blood is shunted to the brain and heart. Treatment includes:

- Immediate establishment of airway, breathing and circulation (ABCs).
- NG tube and gastric decompression to reduce risk of aspiration.
- Neurological evaluation.
- Pulmonary management includes monitoring for ≥72 hours for respiratory deterioration. Ventilation may need positive-end expiratory pressure (PEEP), but this poses danger to cardiac output and can cause barotrauma, so use should be limited.
- In patients that are symptomatic but do not yet need intubation, use supplemental oxygen to keep $SpO_2 > 94\%$.
- Monitoring of cardiac output and function.
- Neurological care to reduce cerebral edema and increased intracranial pressure, and prevent secondary injury.
- Rewarming if necessary (0.5 to 1°C/hr).

AIR LEAK SYNDROMES

Air leak syndromes may result in significant respiratory distress. Leaks may occur spontaneously or secondary to some type of trauma (accidental, mechanical, iatrogenic) or disease. As pressure increases inside alveoli, the alveolar wall pulls away from the perivascular sheath and subsequent alveolar rupture allows air to follow the perivascular planes and flow into adjacent areas. There are two categories

- **Pneumothorax:**
  - Air in the pleural space causes a lung to collapse.
- **Barotrauma/volutrauma** with air in the interstitial space (usually resolve over time):
  - Pneumoperitoneum is air in the peritoneal area, including the abdomen and occasionally the scrotal sac of male infants.
  - Pneumomediastinum is air in the mediastinal area between the lungs.
  - Pneumopericardium is air in the pericardial sac that surrounds the heart.
  - Subcutaneous emphysema is air in the subcutaneous tissue planes of the chest wall.
  - Pulmonary interstitial emphysema (PIE) is air trapped in the interstitium between the alveoli.

PNEUMOTHORAX

Pneumothorax occurs when there is a leak of air into the pleural space, resulting in complete or partial collapse of a lung:

- **Symptoms:** Vary widely depending on the cause and degree of the pneumothorax and whether or not there is underlying disease: Acute pleuritic pain (95%), usually on the affected side, decreased breath sounds, *Tension pneumothorax*: tracheal deviation and hemodynamic compromise.
- **Diagnosis:** Clinical findings. Radiograph: 6-foot upright posterior-anterior. Ultrasound may detect traumatic pneumothorax.
- **Treatment:** Chest-tube thoracostomy with underwater seal drainage is the most common treatment for all types of pneumothorax.
  - Tension pneumothorax: Immediate needle decompression and chest tube thoracostomy.
  - Small pneumothorax, patient stable: Oxygen administration and observation for 3-6 hours. If no increase shown on repeat x-ray, patient may be discharged with another x-ray in 24 hours.
  - Primary spontaneous pneumothorax: catheter aspiration or chest tube thoracostomy.

FOREIGN BODY ASPIRATION

Foreign body aspiration can cause obstruction of the pharynx, larynx or trachea, leading to acute dyspnea or asphyxiation and the object may be drawn distally into the bronchial tree. With adults, most foreign bodies migrate more readily down the right bronchus. Food is the most frequently aspirated, but other small objects, such as coins or needles, may also be aspirated. Sometimes the object causes swelling, ulceration, and general inflammation that hampers removal.

Symptoms:

- *Initial:* Severe coughing, gagging, sternal retraction, wheezing. Objects in the larynx may cause inability to breathe or speak and lead to respiratory arrest. Objects in the bronchus cause cough, dyspnea, and wheezing.
- *Delayed:* Hours, days, or weeks later, an undetected aspirant may cause an infection distal to the aspirated material. Symptoms depend on the area and extent of the infection.

Treatment:

- Removal with laryngoscopy or bronchoscopy (rigid is often better than flexible).
- Antibiotic therapy for secondary infection.
- Surgical bronchotomy (rarely required).
- Symptomatic support.

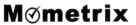

ACUTE PULMONARY EMBOLISM

Acute pulmonary embolism occurs when a pulmonary artery or arteriole is blocked, cutting off blood supply to the pulmonary vessels and subsequent oxygenation of the blood. While most pulmonary emboli are from thrombus formation, other causes may be air, fat, or septic embolus (from bacterial invasion of a thrombus). Common originating sites for thrombus formation are the deep veins in the legs, the pelvic veins, and the right atrium. Causes include stasis related to damage to endothelial wall and changes in blood coagulation factors. Atrial fibrillation poses a serious risk because blood pools in the right atrium, forming clots that travel directly through the right ventricle to the lungs. The obstruction of the artery/arteriole causes an increase in alveolar dead space in which there is ventilation but impairment of gas exchange because of the ventilation/perfusion mismatching or intrapulmonary shunting. This results in hypoxia, hypercapnia, and the release of mediators that cause bronchoconstriction. If more than 50% of the vascular bed becomes excluded, pulmonary hypertension occurs.

SYMPTOMS AND DIAGNOSIS

Clinical manifestations of **acute pulmonary embolism** (PE) vary according to the size of the embolus and the area of occlusion.

Symptoms:

- Dyspnea with tachypnea.
- Cyanosis; may turn grey/blue from nipple line up (massive PE)
- Anxiety and restlessness – "feeling of doom"
- Chest pain, tachycardia – may progress to arrhythmias (PEA)
- Fever.
- Rales.
- Cough (sometimes with hemoptysis).
- Hemodynamic instability.

Diagnostic tests:

- ABG analysis may show hypoxemia (Decreased PaO_2), hypocarbia (Decreased $PaCO_2$) and respiratory alkalosis (Increased pH).
- D-dimer (will show elevation with PE).
- ECG may show sinus tachycardia or other abnormalities.
- Echocardiogram can show emboli in the central arteries and can assess the hemodynamic status of the right side of the heart.
- Spiral CT may provide definitive diagnosis.
- V/Q scintigraphy can confirm diagnosis.
- Pulmonary angiograms also can confirm diagnosis.

MEDICAL MANAGEMENT

Medical management of **pulmonary embolism** starts with preventive measures for those at risk, including leg exercises, elastic compression stockings, and anticoagulation therapy. Most pulmonary emboli present as medical emergencies, so the immediate task is to stabilize the patient. Medical management may include:

- **Oxygen** to relieve hypoxemia.
- **Intravenous infusions:** Dobutamine (Dobutrex®) or dopamine (Intropin®) to relieve hypotension.
- **Cardiac monitoring** for dysrhythmias and issues due to right sided heart failure.

31

- **Medications** as indicated: digitalis glycosides, diuretic, and antiarrhythmics.
- Intubation and mechanical ventilation may be required.
- **Analgesia** (such as morphine sulfate) or sedation to relieve anxiety.
- **Anticoagulants** to prevent recurrence (although it will not dissolve clots already present), including heparin and warfarin (Coumadin®).
- **Placement of percutaneous venous filter** (Greenfield) in the inferior vena cava to prevent further emboli from entering the lungs may be done if anticoagulation therapy is contraindicated.
- **Thrombolytic therapy,** recombinant tissue-type plasminogen activator (rt-PA) or streptokinase, for those severely compromised, but these treatments have limited success and pose the danger of bleeding.

ARDS

Acute lung injury (ALI) comprises a syndrome of respiratory distress culminating in **acute respiratory distress syndrome (ARDS).** ARDS is characterized by damage to the vascular endothelium and an increase in the permeability of the alveolar–capillary membrane when damage to the lung results from toxic substances (e.g., gastric fluids, bacteria, chemicals, toxins emitted by neutrophils as part of the inflammatory-mediated response); these substances reduce surfactant and cause pulmonary edema as the alveoli fill with blood and protein-rich fluid and then collapse (atelectasis). This decrease in surfactant also leads to decreased lung compliance (sometimes referred to as stiffening). The fluid in the alveoli becomes a medium for infection. Because there is neither adequate ventilation nor perfusion, the result is increasing hypoxemia and tachypnea as the body tries to compensate to maintain a normal partial pressure of carbon dioxide. Symptoms are characterized by respiratory distress within 72 hours of surgery or a serious injury to a person with otherwise normal lungs and no cardiac disorder. Untreated, the condition results in respiratory failure, MODS, and a mortality rate of 5-30%. Symptoms: #1 – refractory hypoxemia (hypoxemia not responding to increasing levels of oxygen), crackling rales/wheezing in lungs, ↓ in pulmonary compliance which results in ↑ tachypnea with expiratory grunting, cyanosis/skin mottling, hypotension and tachycardia, symptoms associated with volume overload are missing (3rd heart sound or JVD), respiratory alkalosis initially but replaced as the disease progresses with hypercarbia and respiratory acidosis, and normal X-ray initially but then diffuse infiltrates in both lungs, but the heart and vessels appear normal.

VENTILATOR MANAGEMENT

Ventilator management in acute respiratory distress sydnrome includes:

- O_2 therapy by nasal prongs/cannula or mask may be sufficient in very mild cases to maintain oxygen saturation above 90%. Oxygen should be administered at 100% because of the mismatch between ventilation (V) and perfusion (Q), which can result in hypoxia on position change.
- ARDS oxygenation goal is PaO_2 55-80 mmHg or SpO_2 88-95%.
- Many times endotracheal intubation may be needed if SpO_2 falls or CO_2 levels rise.
- The ARDS Network recommends low tidal volumes (6 mL/kg) and higher PEEP (12 cm H_2O or more).
- The low tidal volume ventilation described above is referred to as lung protective ventilation, and it has been shown to reduce mortality in patients with ARDS.
- For patients with severe ARDS, trials placing patient in prone position 18-24 hours/day with chest and pelvis supported and abdomen unsupported allows the diaphragm to move posteriorly, increasing functional residual capacity (FRC) in many patients.

MANAGEMENT

The management of **acute respiratory distress syndrome (ARDS)** involves providing adequate gas exchange and preventing further damage to the lung from forced ventilation. *Treatment* includes:

- Corticosteroids (may increase mortality rates in some patient populations, though this is the most common given), nitrous oxide, inhaled surfactant, and anti-inflammatory medications.
- Treatment of the underlying condition is the only proven treatment, especially identifying and treating with appropriate antibiotics any infection, as sepsis is most common etiology for ARDS, but prophylactic antibiotics are not indicated.
- Conservative fluid management is indicated to reduce days on the ventilator, but does not reduce overall mortality.

Pharmacologic preventive care: enoxaparin 40 mg subcutaneously QD, sucralfate 1 g NGT four times daily or omeprazole 40 mg IV QD, and enteral nutrition support within 24 hours of ICU admission or intubation.

ACUTE RESPIRATORY FAILURE

The **cardinal signs of respiratory failure** include:

- Tachypnea.
- Tachycardia.
- Anxiety and restlessness.
- Diaphoresis.

Symptoms may vary according to the cause. An obstruction may cause more obvious respiratory symptoms than other disorders. Early signs may include changes in the depth and pattern of respirations with flaring nares, sternal retractions, expiratory grunting, wheezing, and extended expiration as the body tries to compensate for hypoxemia and increasing levels of carbon dioxide. Cyanosis may be evident. Central nervous depression, with alterations in consciousness occurs with decreased perfusion to the brain. As the hypoxemia worsens, cardiac arrhythmias, including bradycardia, may occur with either hypotension or hypertension. Dyspnea becomes more pronounced with depressed respirations. Eventually stupor, coma, and death can occur if the condition is not reversed.

HYPOXEMIC AND HYPERCAPNIC RESPIRATORY FAILURE

Hypoxemic respiratory failure occurs suddenly when gaseous exchange of oxygen for carbon dioxide cannot keep up with demand for oxygen or production of carbon dioxide:

- PaO_2 <60 mm Hg
- $PaCO_2$ >40 mm Hg
- Arterial pH <7.35

Hypoxemic respiratory failure can be the result of low inhaled oxygen, as at high elevations or with smoke inhalation. The following ventilatory mechanisms may be involved:

- Alveolar hypotension
- Ventilation-perfusion mismatch (the most common cause)
- Intrapulmonary shunts
- Diffusion impairment

Hypercapnic respiratory failure results from an increase in $PaCO_2$ >45-50 mm Hg associated with respiratory acidosis and may include:

- Reduction in minute ventilation, total volume of gas ventilated in one minute (often related to neurological, muscle, or chest wall disorders, drug overdoses, obstruction of upper airway.)
- Increased dead space with wasted ventilation (related to lung disease or disorders of chest wall, such as scoliosis).
- Increased production of CO_2 (usually related to infection, burns, or other causes of hypermetabolism).

MANAGEMENT OF THORACIC TRAUMA
FRACTURED RIBS

Fractured ribs are usually the result of severe trauma, such as blunt force from a motor vehicle accident or physical abuse. Underlying injuries should be expected according to the area of fractures:

- Upper 2 ribs: Injuries to trachea, bronchi, or great vessels.
- Right-sided ≥rib 8: Trauma to liver.
- Left-sided ≥ rib 8: Trauma to spleen.

Pain, often localized or experienced on respirations or compression of chest way may be the primary symptom of rib fractures, resulting in shallow breathing that can lead to atelectasis or pneumonia.

Diagnosis: Chest x-ray or CT scan.

Treatment is primarily supportive as rib fractures usually heal in about 6 weeks. However, preventing pulmonary complications (pneumothorax, hemothorax) often necessitates adequate pain control. Underlying injuries are treated according to the type and degree of injury:

- Supplemental oxygen.
- Analgesia may include NSAIDs, intercostal nerve blocks, and narcotics.
- Pulmonary physiotherapy.
- Rib Belts.
- Surgical fixation (ORIF) is usually done only in those requiring thoracotomy for underlying injuries.
- Splinting.

FLAIL CHEST

Flail chest is a more common injury in adults and older teens than children. It occurs when at least 3 adjacent ribs are fractured, both anteriorly and posteriorly, so that they float free of the rib cage. There may be variations, such as the sternum floating with ribs fractured on both sides. Flail chest results in a failure of the chest wall to support changes in intrathoracic pressure so that there paradoxical respirations occur with the flail area contracting on inspiration and expanding on expiration. The lungs are not able to expand properly, decreasing ventilation, but the degree of respiratory distress may relate to injury to underlying structures more than the flail chest alone.

Treatment:

- Initial stabilization with tape, one side only, don't wrap chest.
- Analgesia for pain relief.
- Respiratory physiotherapy to prevent atelectasis.

- Mechanical ventilation is usually not indicated unless needed for underlying injuries.
- Surgical fixation is usually done only in those requiring thoracotomy for underlying injuries.

HEMOTHORAX

Hemothorax occurs with bleeding into the pleural space, usually from major vascular injury such as tears in intercostal vessels, lacerations of great vessels, or trauma to lung parenchyma. A small bleed may be self-limiting and seal, but a tear in a large vessel can result in massive bleeding, followed quickly by hypovolemic shock. The pressure from the blood may result in inability of the lung to ventilate and a mediastinal shift. Often a hemothorax occurs with a pneumothorax, especially in severe chest trauma. Further symptoms include severe respiratory distress, decreased breath sounds, and dullness on auscultation. Treatment includes placement of a chest tube to drain the hemothorax, but with large volumes, the pressure may be preventing exsanguination, which can occur abruptly as the blood drains and pressure is reduced, so a large bore intravenous line should be in place before placement of the chest tube and typed and cross-matched blood immediately available. Autotransfusion may be used, contraindicated if wound is older than three hours, possibility of bowel/stomach contamination, liver failure, and malignancy. Thoracotomy may be indicated after chest tube insertion if there is still hemodynamic instability, tension hemothorax, more than 1500 mL blood initially on insertion, or bleeding continues at a rate of >300 ml/hr.

ABDOMINAL PENETRATING INJURIES

GUNSHOT AND STAB WOUNDS

Penetrating abdominal wounds are almost always related to gunshot wounds (high energy) or knife assaults (low energy stab wounds) and may involve internal injury to multiple organs including intestines liver, stomach and vascular structures:

- **Gunshot wounds** tend to cause more extensive damage than stab wounds, especially to the colon, liver, spleen and diaphragm. Interior injury may be extensive because the bullet damages tissue and may ricochet off of bone. Hemorrhage and peritonitis are common complications. Between 80% and 95% of patients with abdominal gunshot wounds require surgical repair. Bullet wounds should be counted and each assessed for trajectory and entry and exit wounds (helps to determine if bullet retained).
- **Stab wounds** require immediate surgical exploration if the patient is hemodynamically unstable, there are signs of peritoneal hemorrhage, or evisceration is evident or impending. Intraperitoneal injuries require surgical repair, but more conservative treatment (local wound exploration, antibiotics) may be indicated for extraperitoneal wounds. Stab wounds below the nipple line (anterior) and scapular tip (posterior) increase the risk of injury to internal organs.

SPLENIC INJURIES

The **spleen** is the most frequently injured solid organ in blunt trauma. Injuries to the spleen are the most common because it's not well protected by the rib cage and is very vascular. Symptoms may be very non-specific. Kehr sign (radiating pain in left shoulder) indicates intra-abdominal bleeding and Cullen sign (ecchymosis around umbilicus) indicates hemorrhage from ruptured spleen. Some may have right upper abdominal pain although diffuse abdominal pain often occurs with blood loss, associated with hypotension. **Splenic injuries are classified according to the degree of injury:**

I. Tear in splenic capsules or hematoma.
II. Laceration of parenchyma (<3 cm).
III. Laceration of parenchyma (≥3cm).
IV. Multiple lacerations of parenchyma or burst-type injury.

Treatment: Because removing the spleen increases the risk of life-threatening infections, every effort (bed rest, transfusion, reduced activity for at least 8 weeks) is done to avoid surgery (argon gas, fibrin "glue", or therapeutic ultrasound). Lab testing for the absence Howell-Jolly bodies indicates the spleen in functioning properly. If conservative efforts fail (usually occurs in first 72 hours), a splenectomy is performed. After surgery, the patient has an increased risk for infection and thrombosis. Lifetime anticoagulation therapy and vaccinations (combo of pneumonia/meningitis/influenza B vaccine) should be administered.

HEPATIC INJURIES

Hepatic injury is the most common cause of death from abdominal trauma. It is particularly danger as hematoma rupture can occur hours to 6 weeks after the time of injury. Because hepatic injury is often associated with multiple organ damage, symptoms may be non-specific and difficult to diagnose. Therefore, elevation in liver transaminase levels or elevation of right hemidiaphragm on Xray in trauma patients indicates damage that may require further examination. **Liver injuries are classified according to the degree of injury:**

I. Tears in capsule with hematoma.
II. Laceration(s) of parenchyma (<3 cm).
III. Laceration(s) of parenchyma (≥3 cm).
IV. Destruction of 25-75% of lobe from burst injury.
V. Destruction of >75% of lobe from burst injury.
VI. Avulsion [tearing away].

Hemodynamically stable patients are managed medically, but surgical repair may be necessary if the patient is unstable or bleeding. Hemorrhage is common complication of hepatic injury and may require ligation of hepatic arteries or veins. Treatment often includes intravenous fluids for fluid volume deficit as well as blood products (plasma, platelets) for coagulopathies. Surgical or angiographic embolization of the tear may be indicated in severe injury.

COMPARTMENT SYNDROME

Abdominal trauma with pronounced shock increases risk of **compartment syndrome**, in which the pressure in the abdomen increases to the point of acute ischemia and anoxia of the tissues. Causes include edema of the intestines (trauma/surgical manipulation), reduced expansion of abdominal cavity (burns), hemorrhage, and capillary leakage after excessive fluid resuscitation.

- **Signs/Symptoms:** increased airway pressures and acute respiratory distress syndrome, decreased U/O, and cerebral edema.
- **Diagnosis:** increased intra-abdominal pressure (>20 cmH$_2$O), measured by Foley catheter or NG tube with pressure transducer or water-column manometry; ↑ CVP and ICP, ↓ CO and GFR.
- **Treatment:**

  o Medications: Sudden release of pressure and reperfusion may cause acidosis, hyperkalemia, vasodilation, and cardiac arrest. The patient should be given crystalloid solutions before decompression. Treatment may also include milrinone, dopamine, and mannitol.
  o Surgical decompression
  o Prevention - If risk for compartment syndrome exists, the wound should not be closed, but left open and covered with a sterile dressing. Negative-pressure wound therapy may be used to decrease risk.

ACUTE GASTROINTESTINAL HEMORRHAGE

Gastrointestinal (GI) hemorrhage may occur in the upper or lower gastrointestinal track. The primary cause (50-70%) of GI hemorrhage is gastric and duodenal ulcers, generally caused by stress, NSAIDs or infection with *Helicobacter pylori.*

- **Symptoms:** abdominal pain and distention, coffee-ground emesis/ hematemesis, bloody or tarry stools, hypotension with tachycardia.
- **Diagnosis:** stool occult blood (Guaiac test), EGD, colonoscopy, GI Bleed scan.
- **Treatment:**

  - Medications: Fluid replacement with blood transfusions if necessary, antibiotic therapy for *Helicobacter pylori,* continuous pantoprazole IV to prevent further irritation.
  - Endoscopic thermal therapy to cauterize or injection therapy (hypertonic saline, epinephrine, ethanol) to cause vasoconstriction.
  - Arteriography with intraarterial infusion of vasopressin and/or embolizing agents, such as stainless-steel coils, platinum micro coils, or Gelfoam pledgets.
  - Vagotomy and pyloroplasty if bleeding persists.
  - Prevention: prophylactic medications (pantoprazole [Protonix] IV is common).

BOWEL OBSTRUCTION AND INFARCTION

Bowel obstruction occurs when there is a mechanical obstruction of the passage of intestinal contents because of constriction of the lumen, occlusion of the lumen, adhesion formation, or lack of muscular contractions (paralytic ileus). Symptoms include abdominal pain, rigidity, and distention, n/v, dehydration, constipation, and respiratory distress from the diaphragm pushing against the pleural cavity, sepsis and shock. Treatment includes strict NPO, insertion of naso/orogastric tube, IV fluids and careful monitoring; may correct spontaneously, severe obstruction requires surgery.

Bowel infarction is ischemia of the intestines related to severely restricted blood supply. It can be the result of a number of different conditions, such as strangulated bowel or occlusion of arteries of the mesentery, and may follow untreated bowel obstruction. People present with acute abdomen (see card on compartment syndrome) and shock, and mortality rates are very high even with resection of infarcted bowel. Treatment includes replacing volume, correcting the underlying issue, improving blood flow to the mesentery, insertion of NGT, and/or surgery.

INTESTINAL PERFORATION

Intestinal perforation is a partial or complete tear in the intestinal wall, leaking intestinal contents into the peritoneum. Causes include trauma, NSAIDs (elderly, patients with diverticulitis), acute appendicitis, PUD, iatrogenic (laparoscopy, endoscopy, colonoscopy, radiotherapy), bacterial infections, IBS, and ingestion of toxic substances (acids), trauma or foreign bodies (toothpicks). The danger posed by infection after perforation varies depending upon the site. The stomach and proximal portions of the small intestine have little bacteria, but the distal portion of the small intestine contains aerobic bacteria, such as *E. coli,* as well as anaerobic bacteria.

- **Signs/Symptoms:** (appear within 24-48 hours): abdominal pain and distention and rigidity, fever, guarding and rebound tenderness, tachycardia, dyspnea, absent bowel sounds/paralytic ileus with nausea and vomiting; Sepsis and abscess or fistula formation can occur.
- **Diagnosis:** Labs - ↑ WBC; lactic acid and pH change as late signs. X-ray and CT will show free air in abdominal cavity.
- **Treatment:**

- o Prompt antibiotic therapy, and surgical repair with peritoneal lavage.
- o The abdominal wound may be left open to heal by secondary intention and to prevent compartment syndrome
- o See Peritonitis card.

DIAPHRAGMATIC RUPTURE

Diaphragmatic rupture most often results from blunt trauma associated with motor vehicle accident or fall from height resulting in sudden increase in intraabdominal pressure that causes muscle tearing. With blunt trauma, rupture occurs on the left side in 65% to 80% of cases. However, a diaphragmatic rupture can also result from penetrating trauma, such as stab or gunshot wounds. Penetrating wounds are usually smaller initially and may be overlooked but may enlarge over time. Risk factors for diaphragmatic rupture include direct trauma to upper abdomen, severe trauma to chest with fractured lower ribs, and penetrating injuries to upper abdomen or chest. Patients may complain of shortness of breath and pain, but these may not be reliable indicators because other injuries are often present. Diagnosis is per examination and laparotomy. Chest x-ray and CT may not show injury. Surgical repair is required as the muscle will not heal spontaneously and internal organs may herniate.

ACUTE KIDNEY INJURY (AKI)

Acute kidney injury (previously known as acute renal failure) is an acute disruption of kidney function that results in decreased renal perfusion, a decrease in glomerular filtration rate and a buildup of metabolic waste products (azotemia). Azotemia is the accumulation of urea, creatinine and other nitrogen containing end products into the bloodstream. The regulation of fluid volume, electrolyte balance and acid base balance is also affected. The causes of acute kidney injury are divided into pre-renal (caused by a decrease in perfusion), intrarenal or intrinsic (occurring within the kidney) and post-renal (caused by the inadequate drainage of urine). Acute kidney injury is common in hospitalized patients and even more commonly in critically ill patients, carrying a mortality rate of 50-80%. Risk factors for acute kidney injury include advanced age, the presence of co-morbid conditions, pre-existing kidney disease and a diagnosis of sepsis.

- **Signs and symptoms**: malaise, fatigue, lethargy, confusion, weakness, change in urine color, change in urine volume and flank pain.
- **Diagnosis**: urinalysis, serum BUN and creatinine levels, renal ultrasound, CT or MRI and renal biopsy.
- **Treatment**: The treatment of acute kidney injury is based on the underlying cause. Treatment options may include fluid and electrolyte replacement, diuretic therapy, fluid restriction, renal diet, and low dose dopamine to increase renal perfusion. Hemodialysis may also be necessary in patients with acute kidney injury.

OBSTETRICAL COMPLICATIONS ASSOCIATED WITH TRAUMATIC EVENTS

Obstetrical complications associated with trauma include:

- **Motor vehicle accident:** Account for up to 80% of trauma with pregnancy and may result in preterm contractions (up to 40% of trauma patients), preterm birth, placental abruption, fetal mortality, and fetomaternal hemorrhage. Fetomaternal hemorrhage is especially a concern with Rh- mothers, who should receive 300 mcg of Rh-immune globulin (RhoGAM®) within 72 hours of trauma and additional 300 mcg for every 30 mL of estimated fetal blood in maternal circulation. Shearing injuries and placental abruption may result in disseminated intravascular coagulopathy (DIC) because of amniotic fluid embolism. Uterine rupture, while rare, may occur.
- **Asphyxia:** Lack of oxygen can result in hypoxemia and neurological compromise in both the woman and the fetus.

- **Abuse:** The effects of abuse vary according to the type and severity of abuse. Physical abuse, such as hitting or kicking the pregnant woman may result in problems similar to those associated with motor vehicle accidents, including fetal mortality, preterm birth, and uterine rupture. Additionally, the abused woman may not have had adequate prenatal care, increasing risks to the fetus.

INTRAPARTAL AND POST-PARTAL HEMORRHAGE

Intrapartal hemorrhage often occurs because of placenta previa or abruptio placentae or disseminated intravascular coagulation (which may be triggered by release of tissue thromboplastin with abruptio placentae or with a dead fetus). **Post-partal hemorrhage** is blood loss greater than 500 mL following vaginal birth or greater than 1000 mL following Cesarean, or saturation of more than one peri-pad in 15 minutes. A drop in hematocrit of 10% or more may also indicate hemorrhage but may not be accurate with hemorrhage. Hemorrhage:

- **Early postpartum**: Occurs within 24 hours of childbirth and up to 90% is caused by uterine atony, which is often associated with overdistention (multiple gestations, large infant, hydramnios) or weak muscles (multiparity). Induced or precipitous labor increases risk. Early hemorrhage may also be caused by trauma (lacerations and hematomas).
- **Late postpartum**: Occurs more than 24 hours (often up to 6 to 14 days) after childbirth and usually results from subinvolution of uterus or retained placental fragments.

CAUSES OF HEMORRHAGIC COMPLICATIONS DURING PREGNANCY

Hemorrhage during pregnancy puts both fetus and mother at risk of death from hypoxia. Loss of blood predisposes the mother to anemia and infection, and the fetus to premature birth. Placental abruption and uterine rupture are the main causes of hemorrhage resulting in maternal and fetal death. Spontaneous abortion can cause bleeding early in a pregnancy. Ectopic pregnancy is another cause of bleeding early in pregnancy. Placental previa also can result in bleeding early, and can complicate delivery, resulting in the need for a cesarean section. Vasa previa, a condition in which umbilical arteries and veins are in an abnormal position at the opening of the uterus, can result in vessel rupture during a spontaneous rupture of membranes or an artificial amniotomy and rapid fetus demise from fetal hemorrhage.

POSTPARTAL HEMORRHAGE

Following delivery, the nurse must monitor the woman carefully for increased bleeding, severe pain, tachycardia, and uncontracted uterus, as these signs may indicate **postpartal hemorrhage**. The nurse must massage the fundus and apply firm but gentle fundal pressure only to the contracted uterus to express clots as applying pressure to an uncontracted uterus may result in increased hemorrhage and uterine inversion. The nurse should also relieve a distended bladder, which can prevent uterine contraction. The patient may need IV oxytocin or bimanual compression of the uterus to control bleeding. If bleeding is caused by trauma, surgical repair is needed. **Balloon tamponade** may be needed to control bleeding. Specially designed catheters have a balloon (usually 500 mL capacity) that is inflated with NS after insertion into the uterus. Many balloon catheters are bi-luminal so that blood can drain and be measured to determine if the pressure applied by the balloon is controlling bleeding. The balloon catheter should control bleeding within 5 to 15 minutes.

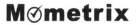

Extremity and Wounds

COMPARTMENT SYNDROME

Compartment syndrome occurs when there is an increase in the amount of pressure within a grouping of muscles, nerves and blood vessels resulting in compromised blood flow to muscles and nerves. If left untreated, tissue ischemia and eventual tissue death will occur. Compartment syndrome most often occurs after a fracture, particularly a long bone fracture, but can also occur with crushing syndrome and rhabdomyolysis.. Risk factors include lower extremity trauma, massive tissue injury, venous obstruction, the use of certain medications (anticoagulants), burns and compressive dressings or casts. Compartment syndrome can affect the hand, forearm, upper arm, abdomen and lower extremities. It can be acute or chronic in nature with acute compartment syndrome requiring immediate intervention.

- **Signs and symptoms**: Intense pain, decreased sensation and paresthesia, firmness at the affected site, swelling and tightness at the affected site, pallor and pulselessness (late signs).
- **Diagnosis**: Physical assessment and the measurement of intra-compartmental pressures.
- **Treatment**: The goal of treatment in compartment syndrome is decompression and the restoration of perfusion to the affected area. Surgical fasciotomy is often indicated to relieve pressure and prevent tissue death. Fasciotomy involves the opening of the skin and muscle fascia to release the pressure within the compartment and restore blood flow to the area.
- **Prevention**: Leave large abdominal wounds open to drain, delay casting on affected extremities /use flexible casts. Watch circumferential burns closely, frequent neurovascular checks on those at risk.

RHABDOMYOLYSIS

Rhabdomyolysis occurs when damage of the cells of the skeletal muscles causes the release of toxins from injured cells into the bloodstream. Rhabdomyolysis may be caused by trauma, tissue ischemia, infection, certain medications (statins, selective serotonin reuptake inhibitors, lithium and antihistamines), sepsis, immobilization, extraordinary physical exertion, myopathies and cocaine or alcohol abuse. Additionally, rhabdomyolysis may occur with exposure to certain toxins such as snake/insect venoms or mushroom poisoning. In rare circumstances, the identifiable cause cannot be determined. The most serious complication of rhabdomyolysis is renal failure. Rhabdomyolysis may be life threatening. Early recognition and treatment is critical to avoid serious complications and for patients to make a full recovery.

- **Signs and symptoms**: electrolyte imbalance, muscle pain and weakness, fever, tachycardia, dehydration, fatigue, lethargy, hypotension and metabolic acidosis. Dark, reddish-brown urine may occur due to the presence of myoglobin released from the muscles and excreted into the urine.
- **Diagnosis**: laboratory studies such as creatinine kinase (CK) level, metabolic panel, urinalysis and blood gases.
- **Treatment**: The treatment of rhabdomyolysis includes fluid administration to eliminate toxins and prevent renal failure. Bicarbonate may be administered to correct metabolic acidosis. Mannitol or dopamine may be administered to increase renal perfusion. Electrolyte replacement may also be indicated. In severe cases, emergency dialysis may be necessary.

CARE OF TRAUMATIC WOUNDS

Traumatic wounds include cuts, punctures, lacerations, force trauma, gunshot wounds, bites, abrasions, crush injuries, degloving injuries and contusions. Trauma wounds can vary in severity and may be associated with serious underlying injuries. Once the patient is stabilized, wound management is initiated and should include thorough wound cleansing and debridement with removal of any foreign objects or materials. Irrigation and debridement are critical steps in minimizing the risk of infection. Signs and symptoms include bleeding, pain, erythema and edema. With severe traumatic injury patients may experience signs of hemorrhagic shock including heavy bleeding, loss of consciousness, tachypnea, tachycardia, hypotension, decreased urinary output and pallor.

Treatment of traumatic wounds is dependent on the location and severity of the wound. Treatment options may include irrigation and debridement, foreign body removal, wound closure including sutures, staples or fibrin glue, antibiotics, prophylactic Tetanus injection, and fasciotomy.

INFLAMMATORY PHASE OF WOUND HEALING

Immediately after tissue injury (within 5 to 10 minutes), epinephrine, norepinephrine, thromboxane, and prostaglandins are released; these mediators initiate vasoconstriction, which functions to control any hemorrhage in the area. This is followed by endothelial retraction, which exposes collagen on the subendothelium. Platelets attach to the collagen using fibrinogen, and the attached platelets then attract other platelets to form a platelet plug; this process is called platelet adhesion and aggregation. The aggregated platelets, which are now activated, release serotonin, histamine, and platelet-derived growth factor (PDGF) to initiate the coagulation cascade. The end result of the cascade is the activation of thrombin, which serves 2 purposes: to convert fibrinogen to fibrin, and to increase vascular permeability. The increase in permeability allows inflammatory cells to move from the bloodstream into the injured tissue. Neutrophils dominate the inflammatory picture in the early stages, and are later replaced by monocytes and tissue macrophages, which clean up the debris. Vasodilation increases the blood flow to the area to deliver more cells, fluid, and nutrients, and contributes to tissue edema.

MATURATION PHASE OF WOUND HEALING

The **maturation phase of wound healing** consists mostly of the remodeling of collagen in the wound. Collagen remodeling is a somewhat complex process in which collagen is both removed and synthesized. The removal of old collagen from the wound occurs as a result of various enzymes, including collagenases and matrix metalloproteinases. During this remodeling process, type III collagen is slowly replaced by type I collagen, and proteoglycans replace hyaluronic acid, while water is reabsorbed from the area. This eliminates spaces between collagen fibers, and promotes a more orderly distribution of fibers, thus reducing the size of the scar over time.

PROLIFERATIVE PHASE OF WOUND HEALING

The **proliferative phase of wound healing** begins at the end of the inflammatory phase (there is some overlap), usually within 3 to 5 days after the initial injury. Epithelialization is important; the purpose is to create a new layer of epithelium over the surface of the wound. In simple terms, this is a 2-step process: the epithelial cells proliferate from the edges of the wound and grow toward the center as the clot is dissolved. The epithelial cells secrete enzymes to stimulate the formation of plasmin, which slowly dissolves the clot as the epithelial layer is forming. Under the epithelial surface, fibroblasts are synthesizing and depositing collagen and elastin to restore the tissue to its pre-injured state. New blood vessels are formed during this time (a process called angiogenesis) to deliver enzymes, macrophages, and other nutrients and cells. The blood vessels disappear as the need for them decreases. At the end of this phase, the wound tightens as the cells at the periphery contract.

HIGH ENERGY JOINT INJURIES

Low energy injuries include those that occur as a result of a fall from standing position or less than one-meter height, but **high energy injuries** include those with greater impact, such as from an automobile accident, fall from greater height, and sports accidents (downhill skiing, ice hockey) as well as gunshot wounds, stab wounds, and blast injuries. High energy injuries are likely to be more severe and may include:

- Fractures, both open and closed.
- Compression fractures.
- Dislocations and fracture-dislocations
- Comminution.
- Strains and sprains, injury to ligaments and tendons.
- Lacerations, bleeding.
- Soft tissue trauma, edema and ecchymosis.
- Shock.

Patients typically have severe pain, and the affected joint may be very unstable with obvious misalignment if fractures or dislocations are present. Older adults are particularly at risk for fractures because of osteoporosis, and healing may be impaired because of chronic disease. With high energy injuries, patients also have greater risk of complications, such as fat embolism, hemorrhage, pulmonary embolism, compartment syndrome, infection, neurological damage, infection, avascular necrosis, and mal-union, delayed union, or non-union.

IMMEDIATE INTERVENTIONS FOR TRAUMATIC AMPUTATION

Amputations may be partial or complete. The amputated limb should be treated initially as though it could be reattached or revascularized. Single digits, except the thumb, are often not reattached. Initial treatment includes stabilizing patient and stopping bleeding by applying a proximal blood pressure cuff proximal to injury 30 mm Hg above systolic for <30 minutes. Instruments, such as clamps and hemostats, should be avoided. Other treatment includes:

- Tetanus prophylaxis.
- Analgesia.
- Prophylactic antibiotics may be needed.
- Irrigation of stump with NS (not antiseptics) if contaminated.
- Splint and elevate stump, with saline-moistened sterile dressing in place.
- Neurovascular examinations of stump.

The Allen test should be done to determine arterial injury if digits are amputated. In the Allen test, both the radial and ulnar artery are compressed and the patient is asked to clench the hand repeatedly until it blanches, and then one artery is released, and the tissue on that side should flush. Then the test is repeated again, releasing the other artery.

CARE OF AMPUTATED PART PRIOR TO REATTACHMENT OR REVASCULARIZATION

The **amputated part** should be cooled to 4°C to extend the time of viability and decrease damage from ischemia. (Single digits and lower limbs are not usually reattached, but the limbs should be treated as though they will until determination is made, especially for children.) The part should be reattached within 6 hours if possible but up to 24 hours if properly cooled. Initial care of amputated part includes:

- Removal of jewelry.
- Irrigation with NS to remove debris or contamination.
- Part stored wrapped in saline moistened dressing but NOT immersed in saline or hypotonic solution.

42

- Minimal handling to prevent tissue damage.
- Cool by placing wrapped part in sealed plastic bag and immersing the bag in ice water (1:1 ice to water). Avoid freezing the part.

If the amputation is partial, treatment is similar but NS wrapped part is splinted and ice packs or commercial cold packs are applied over area that is devascularized.

PELVIC FRACTURES

Pelvic fractures may be fairly benign or seriously life threatening, depending on the degree and type of fracture. They most often result from high-speed trauma related to vehicular accidents or skiing accidents:

- **Open book**: Pelvis is pulled apart, usually from frontal injury (may cause severe hemorrhage).
- **Closed book**: Lateral compression occurs from side injury.
- **Vertical shear**: Injury occurs from fall.

Indications of pelvic fracture include localized edema, tenderness, obvious pelvic deformity, abnormal pelvic movement, and abdominal bruising. Associated intra-abdominal injuries and complications are common, including paralytic ileus, hemorrhage, urethral, colon, or bladder laceration. Patients may develop sepsis, peritonitis, fat embolism syndrome, or DVT. Displaced fractures may require open reduction and internal fixation. Treatment usually includes bedrest (up to 6 weeks) with care in handling to prevent further injury. Patients should be turned and moved in accordance with specific physician's orders. Ambulation using walker or crutches may be allowed for non-displaced fractures.

ACETABULAR FRACTURES

Acetabular (hip-socket) fractures occur primarily in young adults with motor vehicle accidents or falls from a height, resulting in impact pressure from the head of the femur to the joint and frequently associated (up to 50% of cases) with other severe injuries, including dislocation (which can lead to avascular necrosis if not promptly reduced). Up to 20% of those with acetabular fractures also have pelvic fractures. The degree of displacement that occurs depends on the amount of force as well as the position of the femur during impact. Acetabular fracture may be classified as posterior-wall, posterior-column, anterior-column, or transverse. Acetabular fractures in children less than 12 years may result in growth arrest. Complications may include sepsis, chondrolysis, and injury to vessels and/or nerves. Post-traumatic arthritis of the joint may develop. Diagnosis is per examination, radiograph, and/or CT with Doppler ultrasound with suspected DVT. Treatment includes emergent closed reduction if necessary, longitudinal skeletal traction, and open reduction and internal fixation (ORIF) for displaced fractures and serious injury (usually delayed for 2 to 3 days because of initial bleeding).

CLOSED FRACTURES AND OPEN FRACTURES

Closed fractures are those in which the damage to the bone and tissue (bleeding, swelling) remains enclosed within intact skin and does not invade any internal cavity. The bones segments are more likely to be aligned although some comminution may have occurred from splintering when the bone breaks. It may be difficult to differentiate a closed fracture from an open fracture if there are abrasions and lacerations over the area of the fractures, but it is closed if there is no continuity between the fracture and the external injury.

Open fractures, on the other hand, cause an external wound and may result from fragments of the fractured bone penetrating the skin or an external force penetrating the skin and bone. Open fractures may also appear closed on the surface but invade a body cavity. Open fractures carry a much higher risk of contamination and infection as well as severe bleeding. The external wounds associated with open fractures may vary in size but even small wounds are considered emergent because of risk of infection.

FAT EMBOLISM AS COMPLICATION OF TRAUMATIC FRACTURE

In instances of **traumatic fracture**, the possibility of **fat embolism** should be considered; this is especially true in fractures involving the long bones (femur, humerus). When the bone is fractured, this allows for some of the fatty marrow contained within the bone to escape. Because the fracture and subsequent trauma to the area surrounding the fracture results in broken vessels, it is possible that the fatty marrow can be introduced into the bloodstream. When this happens, the events are similar to that of a deep venous thrombosis; the fat embolus dislodges from the lumen of the vessel and travels to the lung. When the embolus enters the pulmonary circulation, it eventually blocks blood flow as the caliber of the vessel through which it travels decreases, keeping blood from flowing to the lung tissue. The disruption in blood flow results in inflammation and necrosis of the lung, and eventually pulmonary failure ensues.

OSTEOMYELITIS AS COMPLICATION OF FRACTURE INJURIES

Osteomyelitis is infection of the bone, usually from extension of soft tissue infection (infected ulcer); puncture wound (bone surgery or traumatic injury, such as open fracture) and bloodborne infection. Osteomyelitis is common in the foot with *Pseudomonas* most often in non-diabetics and *Staphylococcus aureus* in diabetics, who are 3 times more likely to develop osteomyelitis. Symptoms vary according to cause. Onset may be sudden if bloodborne with constant throbbing pain. The area may be erythematous and edematous if from adjacent infection, and chronic conditions may exhibit constant or intermittent drainage and pain. Diagnosis includes x-ray, radioisotope bones scans, MRI, and CBC, wound and blood cultures. Treatment includes identifying and treating underlying cause:

- IV antibiotic therapy based on diagnosis is begun around the clock initially and modified with results of culture, usually continuing for 2-3 weeks.
- Supportive measures: Diet high in vitamins and protein, good hydration.
- Immobilization of affected area to reduce pain and prevent fractures.
- Warm wet soaks 20 minutes 4 times daily.
- Referral for surgical debridement as indicated.

CHEMICAL BURNS

Chemical burns may result from contact with acid or alkali substances. The pH ranges from 1 to 14 with 7 neutral and extremely acidic 1 and extremely alkaline 14. Alkali burns tend to be more severe because acid burns denature proteins, resulting in formation of eschar that prevents deeper penetration of the acid. Alkaline burns, however, both denature proteins and hydrolyze fats, allowing for deeper penetration and tissue damage because of liquefaction necrosis. Hydrofluoric acid is similar to alkaline substances in that it also causes liquefaction necrosis. Symptoms vary depending on the substance, strength, and site of injury but often includes severe pain, tissue blistering and sloughing, and bleeding. Initial treatment includes removal of contaminated clothing and copious wound irrigation with water. If substances contain Na, K, Mg, or metallic lithium, then the burn area should be covered with mineral oil rather than irrigated. If hydrofluoric acid, copious water irrigations and soft-tissue injection or IV infusion of calcium gluconate may help reduce pain and tissue destruction. Patients may need fluid resuscitation and skin grafting. Complications include disfigurement, infection, and electrolyte imbalance.

ELECTRICAL BURNS

Electrical injuries result from electricity passing through the body from contact with live wires, lighting strikes, and short-circuiting equipment. Injuries may be high voltage (≥1000 volts) or low voltage (<1000 volts). Electrical injuries can result in extensive subdermal burns. The injury severity correlates with resistance of tissue and current amperage (AC usually causes more damage than DC). Tissue with the highest degree of resistance tends to suffer the most damage with low voltage injury, but high voltage injury can destroy all tissue. Tissue resistance (highest to lowest) include bone >fat >tendons >skin >muscles >vessels > nerves.

- **Low voltage** injuries may cause cardiac dysrhythmias (VF), external burns, tissue damage, fractures and dislocations from muscle contractions, respiratory arrest, or oral burns (children particularly). Treatment includes monitoring and cardiac care as needed, topical antimicrobials, and excision and grafting if necessary.
- **High voltage** injuries may result in additional symptoms of myonecrosis, thrombosis, compartment syndrome, nerve entrapment syndrome. Treatment may include fluid resuscitation, wound debridement, fasciotomy, and amputation, topical antibiotics, systemic antibiotics, and analgesia.

THERMAL BURNS

Thermal burns are caused by heat (hot iron, stove, sun exposure) or fire. Burn injuries begin with the skin but can affect all organs and body systems, especially with a major burn. **Management** of burn injuries must include both wound care and systemic care to avoid complications that can be life threatening. Patients may experience open blistering wounds and severe pain. **Treatment** varies according to severity and may include:

- Establishment of airway and treatment for inhalation injury if necessary.
- Cleansing of burned areas, flushing.
- Debridement of open blisters (no needle aspiration).
- Tetanus immunization if needed.
- Intravenous fluids and electrolytes, based on weight and extent of burn.
- Enteral feedings, usually with small lumen feeding tube into the duodenum.
- NG tube for gastric decompression to prevent aspiration.
- Indwelling catheter to monitor urinary output. Urinary output should be 0.5-2 mL/kg/hr.
- Analgesia for reduction of pain and anxiety.
- Topical (usually silver sulfadiazine) and systemic antibiotics.
- Wound care with removal of eschar and dressings as indicated.
- Skin grafting.

Complications include scarring, disfigurement, contractures, and infection.

INHALATION INJURIES

Inhalation injuries most often result from exposure to smoke in closed spaces, and are often associated with conditions that affect mentation, such as intoxication or head injury. Thermal injuries occur to the upper airway, but inhalation causes injury below the vocal cords. Toxic inhalants can include tissue asphyxiants, pulmonary irritants, and systemic toxins. Patients may suffer from carbon monoxide and hydrogen cyanide poisoning. Symptoms of inhalation injuries include dyspnea with bronchospasm, coma from brain hypoxia (carbon monoxide poisoning), rapid upper airway edema and delayed ($\leq$ 24 hours) lower airway edema. Diagnosis includes clinical examination, ABGs and carboxyhemoglobin levels, pulse oximetry, fiberoptic bronchoscopy, and chest radiograph. Treatments include:

- Humidified oxygen, 100%.
- Evaluation or hyperbaric oxygen therapy (carbon monoxide poisoning).
- β-agonists for bronchospasm, followed by aminophylline if ineffective.
- Endotracheal intubation and mechanical ventilation if indicated by severity of burns or respiratory status.

- Tracheostomy for long-term (>14 days) ventilation.
- Anti-toxin therapy according to inhalant (sodium nitrate or sodium thiosulfate for cyanide).

Complications include permanent damage to respiratory system and neurological compromise from hypoxemia.

MULTISYSTEM COMPLICATIONS OF BURN INJURIES

Burn injuries begin with the skin but can affect all organs and body systems, especially with a major burn:

- **Cardiovascular**: Cardiac output may fall by 50% as capillary permeability increases with vasodilation and fluid leaks from the tissues.
- **Urinary**: Decreased blood flow causes kidneys to increase ADH, which increases oliguria. BUN and creatinine levels increase. Cell destruction may block tubules, and hematuria may result from hemolysis.
- **Pulmonary**: Injury may result from smoke inhalation or (rarely) aspiration of hot liquid. Pulmonary injury is a leading cause of death from burns and is classified according to degree of damage:
  - First: Singed eyebrows and nasal hairs with possible soot in airways and slight edema.
  - Second: (At 24 hours) Stridor, dyspnea, and tachypnea with edema and erythema of upper airway, including area of vocal chords and epiglottis.
  - Third: (At 72 hours) worsening symptoms if not intubated and if intubated, bronchorrhea and tachypnea with edematous, secreting tissue.
- **Neurological**: Encephalopathy may develop from lack of oxygen, decreased blood volume and sepsis. Hallucinations, alterations in consciousness, seizures and coma may result.
- **Gastrointestinal**: Ileus and ulcerations of mucosa often result from poor circulation. Ileus usually clears within 48-72 hours, but if it returns it is often indicative of sepsis.
- **Endocrine/Metabolic:** The sympathetic nervous system stimulates the adrenals to release epinephrine and norepinephrine to increase cardiac output and cortisol for wound healing. The metabolic rate increases markedly. Electrolyte loss occurs with fluid loss from exposed tissue, especially phosphorus, calcium and sodium, with an increase in potassium levels. Electrolyte imbalance can be life-threatening if burns cover >20% of BSA. Glycogen depletion occurs within 12-24 hours and protein breakdown and muscle wasting occurs without sufficient intake of protein.

MANAGEMENT OF BURN INJURIES

Management of burn injuries must include both wound care and systemic care to avoid complications that can be life threatening. Treatment includes:

- Establishment of airway and treatment for inhalation injury as indicated:
  - Supplemental oxygen, incentive spirometry, nasotracheal suctioning.
  - Humidification.
  - Bronchoscopy as needed to evaluate bronchospasm and edema.
  - β-Agonists for bronchospasm, followed by aminophylline if ineffective.
- Intubation and ventilation if there are indications of respiratory failure. This should be done prior to failure. Tracheostomy may be done if ventilation >14 days.
- Intravenous fluids and electrolytes, based on weight and extent of burn. Parkland formula: Fluid replacement (mL) in first 24 hours = (mass in kg) × (body % burned) × 400.
- Enteral feedings, usually with small lumen feeding tube into the duodenum.

46

- NG tube for gastric decompression to prevent aspiration.
- Indwelling catheter to monitor urinary output. Urinary output should be 0.5-2 ml/kg/hr.
- Analgesia for reduction of pain and anxiety.
- Topical and systemic antibiotics.
- Wound care with removal of eschar and dressings as indicated.

Special Considerations

DELIRIUM

Delirium is an acute, sudden, and fluctuating change in consciousness. Delirium occurs in 10-40% of hospitalized older adults and about 80% of patients who are terminally ill. Delirium may result from drugs, infections, hypoxia, trauma, dementia, depression, vision and hearing loss, surgery, alcoholism, untreated pain, fluid/electrolyte imbalance, and malnutrition. If left untreated, delirium greatly increases the risk of morbidity and death.

- **Signs/Symptoms:** Reduced ability to focus/ sustain attention, language and memory disturbances, disorientation, confusion, audiovisual hallucinations, sleep disturbance, and psychomotor activity disorder.
- **Diagnosis:** Patient interview, history/chart/medication review, possible blood tests to identify electrolyte imbalance/abnormalities.
- **Treatment:**
    o Medications: trazodone, lorazepam, haloperidol – though these may make confusion worse in elderly patients
    o Procedures: provide sitter to ensure safety, decreasing dosage of hypnotics and psychotropics, correct underlying cause
    o Prevention: re-orient patient frequently, ensure adequate rest/nutrition, monitor response to medications, and treat infections and dehydration/malnutrition early.

RECOGNITION OF AND TREATMENT FOR AGITATION/DELIRIUM

Agitation is a common occurrence in the critically ill patient. Factors contributing to the development of agitation include drug or alcohol withdrawal, sleep deprivation, hypoxemia, electrolyte or metabolic imbalance, anxiety, pain and adverse drug reactions. Delirium, another common occurrence in the critically ill patient, may also include agitation as a manifestation. A high percentage of critically ill patients develop delirium. Delirium is characterized by changes in cognition that may include disorientation and confusion, disorganized thinking and an altered level of consciousness.

- **Diagnosis**: The physiologic effects of agitation may include increases in heart rate, respiratory rate, blood pressure, intracranial pressure and oxygen consumption. In addition, agitation can contribute to the self-removal of lines or tubes and combative behavior that may result in patient harm.
- **Treatment**: Treatment of agitation involves the identification and correction of causative factors. The use of pharmacologic agents to manage pain, anxiety and agitation are often utilized. Non-pharmacologic interventions including verbal de-escalation (when possible), promoting of normal sleep patterns and relaxation techniques may also be effective. Early identification of signs and symptoms is also critical in the successful management of agitation/delirium.

ASSESSMENT WITH CONFUSION ASSESSMENT METHOD

The **Confusion Assessment Method** is an assessment tool intended to be used by those without psychiatric training in order to assess the progression of delirium in patients. The tool covers 9 factors:

47

some factors have a range of possibilities, and others are rated only as to whether the characteristic is "present", "not present", "uncertain", or "not applicable". The tool also provides room to describe abnormal behavior. Factors indicative of delirium include:

- **Onset**: Acute change in mental status.
- **Attention**: Inattentive, stable or fluctuating.
- **Thinking**: Disorganized, rambling conversation, switching topics, illogical.
- **Level of consciousness:** Altered, ranging from alert to coma.
- **Orientation**: Disoriented (person, place, and time).
- **Memory**: Impaired.
- **Perceptual disturbances:** Hallucinations, illusions.
- **Psychomotor abnormalities:** Agitation (tapping, picking, moving) or retardation (staring, not moving).
- **Sleep-wake cycle:** Awake at night and sleepy in the daytime.

The tool indicates delirium if there is an acute onset, fluctuating inattention, and disorganized thinking OR altered level of consciousness.

PTSD

Patients that experience a traumatic event may re-experience the trauma through distressing thoughts and recollections of the event. In addition, psychological effects of the trauma may include difficulty sleeping, emotional lability and problems with memory and concentration. Patients may also wish to avoid places or activities that remind them of the trauma. These are all characteristics of **post-traumatic stress disorder (PTSD)** and may cause patients extreme distress and significantly impact their quality of life.

- **Signs and symptoms**: nightmares, flashbacks, insomnia, symptoms of hyperarousal including irritability and anxiety, avoidance, and negative thoughts and feelings about oneself and others.
- **Diagnosis**: PTSD is diagnosed through psychological assessment and criteria defined in the Diagnostic and Statistical Manual of Mental Disorders, Fifth Edition (DSM-5).
- **Treatment**: Pharmacologic therapy may be utilized to help control the symptoms of PTSD. Non-pharmacologic therapy options include group and individual/family therapy, cognitive behavioral therapy, and anxiety management / relaxation techniques. Hypnosis may also be utilized.

COGNITIVE ASSESSMENT

Individuals with evidence of dementia, delirium, or short-term memory loss should have cognition assessed. The **mini-mental state exam (MMS)** or the **mini-cog test** are both commonly used. These tests require the individual to carry out specified tasks, and are used as a baseline to determine change in mental status.

MMS:

- Remembering and later repeating the names of 3 common objects.
- Counting backward from 100 by 7s or spelling "world" backward.
- Naming items as the examiner points to them.
- Providing the location of the examiner's office, including city, state, and street address.
- Repeating common phrases.
- Copying a picture of interlocking shapes.
- Following simple 3-part instructions, such a picking up a piece of paper, folding it in half, and placing it on the floor.

A score of ≥24/30 is considered a normal functioning level.

Mini-cog:

- Remembering and later repeating the names of 3 common objects.
- Drawing the face of a clock, including all 12 numbers and the hands, and indicating the time specified by the examiner.

SHOCK
CHARACTERISTICS

There are a number of different types of **shock**, but there are general characteristics that they have in common. In all types of shock, there is a marked decrease in tissue perfusion related to hypotension, so that there is insufficient oxygen delivered to the tissues and, in turn, inadequate removal of cellular waste products, causing injury to tissue:

- Hypotension (systolic below 90 mm Hg). This may be somewhat higher (110 mm Hg) in those who are initially hypertensive.
- Decreased urinary output (<0.5 mL/kg/hr), especially marked in hypovolemic shock
- Metabolic acidosis.
- Peripheral/cutaneous vasoconstriction/vasodilation resulting in cool, clammy skin.
- Alterations in level of consciousness.

Types of Shock:

- **Distributive:** Preload ↓, CO ↑, SVR ↓
- **Cardiogenic:** Preload ↑, CO ↓, SVR ↑
- **Hypovolemic:** Preload ↓, CO ↓, SVR ↑

CARDIOGENIC SHOCK

In **cardiogenic shock**, the heart fails to pump enough blood to provide adequate circulation and oxygen to the body. The primary cause of cardiogenic shock is acute myocardial infarction, especially an anterior wall MI. Other causes include papillary muscle/ ventricular septal rupture, pericarditis/myocarditis, prolonged tachyarrhythmia, and hypotensive medications.

- **Signs/Symptoms**: hypotension, altered mental status secondary to decreased cerebral circulation, oliguria, tachypnea or tachycardia, cool extremities, jugular venous distension and pulmonary edema possible.
- **Diagnosis**: ABGs: metabolic acidosis, hypoxia, hypocapnia; lactic acidosis, BNP, BUN and K ↑; EKG: arrhythmias, specifically SVT/V-tach, Sinus bradycardia, AV block and IVCDs possible; however, may be normal. Arterial Line Values: CI <1.8 L/min, PCWP >18 mm Hg, SBP <90, MAP <60, Increased CVP and PAP
- **Treatment:**
  - Dobutamine IV to increase cardiac contractility;
  - Norepinephrine IV if SBP <70
  - Morphine can be given for pain; while potential for hypotension, it will decrease SNS response and decrease HR and MVO_2
  - Treat underlying cause! (i.e papillary rupture = valve replacement
  - Intra-aortic Balloon Pump (IABP): increases cardiac blood flow
  - Re-vascularization if secondary to acute MI (CABG or PCI)

DISTRIBUTIVE SHOCK

Distributive shock occurs with adequate blood volume but inadequate intravascular volume because of arterial/venous dilation that results in decreased vascular tone and hypoperfusion of internal organs. Cardiac output may be normal or blood may pool, decreasing cardiac output. Distributive shock may result from anaphylactic shock, septic shock, neurogenic shock, and drug ingestions.

Symptoms:

- Hypotension (systolic <90mm Hg or <40mm Hg from normal), tachypnea, tachycardia (>90) (may be lower if patient receiving β-blockers); Hypoxemia.
- Skin initially warm, later hypoperfused.
- Hyper- or hypothermia (>38°C or <36°C).
- Alterations in mentation.
- Decreased urinary output.
- Symptoms related to underlying cause

Treatment:

- Treating underlying cause while stabilizing hemodynamics
- Oxygen with endotracheal intubation if necessary.
- Rapid fluid administration at 0.25-0.5L NS or isotonic crystalloid every 5-10 minutes as needed to 2-3 L.
- Vasoconstrictive and inotropic agents (dopamine, dobutamine, norepinephrine) if necessary, for patients with profound hypotension

NEUROGENIC SHOCK

Neurogenic shock is a type of distributive shock that occurs when there is injury to the CNS from trauma resulting in acute spinal cord injury (from both blunt and penetrating injuries), neurological diseases, drugs, or anesthesia, impairs the autonomic nervous system that controls the cardiovascular system. The degree of symptoms relates to the level of injury with injuries above T1 capable of causing disruption of the entire sympathetic nervous system and lower injuries causing various degrees of disruption. Even incomplete spinal cord injury can cause neurogenic shock.

Symptoms:

- Hypotension and warm dry skin related to lack of vascular tone that results in hypothermia from loss of cutaneous heat.
- Bradycardia is a common but not universal symptom.

Treatment:

- ABCDE (airway, breathing, circulation, disability evaluation, exposure)
- Rapid fluid administration with crystalloid to keep mean arterial pressure at 85-90 mm Hg.
- Placement of pulmonary artery catheter to monitor fluid overload.
- Inotropic agents (dopamine, dobutamine) if fluids don't correct hypotension.
- Atropine for persistent bradycardia.

SEPTIC SHOCK
PATHOLOGY

Septic shock is caused by toxins produced by bacteria and cytokines that the body produces in response to severe infection, resulting in a complex syndrome of disorders. Symptoms are wide-ranging:

- Initial: Hyper- or hypothermia, increased temperature (↑38°C) with chills, tachycardia with increased pulse pressure, tachypnea, alterations in mental status (dullness), hypotension, hyperventilation with respiratory alkalosis (PaCO$_2$ ≤30 mm Hg), increased lactic acid, and unstable BP, and dehydration with increased urinary output.
- Cardiovascular: Myocardial depression and dysrhythmias.
- Respiratory: Acute respiratory distress syndrome (ARDS).
- Renal: acute kidney injury (AKI) with ↓ urinary output and ↑ BUN.
- Hepatic: Jaundice and liver dysfunction with ↑in transaminase, alkaline phosphatase and bilirubin.
- Hematologic: Mild or severe blood loss (from mucosal ulcerations), neutropenia or neutrophilia, decreased platelets, and DIC.
- Endocrine: Hyperglycemia, hypoglycemia (rare).
- Skin: cellulitis, erysipelas, and fasciitis, acrocyanotic and necrotic peripheral lesions.

DIAGNOSIS AND TREATMENT

Septic shock is most common in newborns, those >50, and those who are immunocompromised. There is no specific test to confirm a diagnosis of septic shock, so diagnosis is based on clinical findings and tests that evaluate hematologic, infectious, and metabolic states: Lactic acid, CBC, DIC panel, electrolytes, liver function tests, BUN, creatinine, blood glucose, ABGs, urinalysis, ECG, radiographs, blood and urine cultures. **Treatment** must be aggressive and includes:

- Oxygen and endotracheal intubation as necessary.
- IV access with 2-large bore catheters and central venous line.
- Rapid fluid administration at 0.5L NS or isotonic crystalloid every 5-10 minutes as needed (to 4-6 L).
- Monitoring urinary output to optimal >30mL/hr (>0.5-1mL/kg/hr)
- Inotropic or vasoconstrictive agents (dopamine, dobutamine, norepinephrine) if no response to fluids or fluid overload.
- Empiric IV antibiotic therapy (usually with 2 broad spectrum antibiotics for both gram-positive and gram-negative bacteria) until cultures return and antibiotics may be changed.
- Hemodynamic and laboratory monitoring.
- Removing source of infection (abscess, catheter).

OBSTRUCTIVE SHOCK

Obstructive shock occurs when the preload (diastolic filling of the RV) of the heart is obstructed because of obstruction to the great vessels of the heart (such as from pulmonary embolism). This can also lead to excessive afterload if the flow of blood out of the heart is obstructed (resulting in decreased cardiac output), or with direct compression of the heart, which can occur when blood or air fills the pericardial sac with cardiac tamponade or tension pneumothorax. Other causes include aortic dissection, vena cava syndrome, systemic hypertension, and cardiac lesions. Obstructive shock is often categorized with cardiogenic shock because of similarities. Signs and symptoms of obstructive shock may vary depending on the underlying cause but typically include:

- Decrease in oxygen saturation.
- Hemodynamic instability with hypotension and tachycardia, muffled heart sounds.
- Chest pain.
- Neurological impairment (disorientation, confusion).
- Dyspnea.
- Impaired peripheral circulation (cool extremities, pallor).
- Generalized pallor and cyanosis.

Treatment depends on the cause and may include oxygen, pericardiocentesis, needle thoracostomy or chest tube, and fluid resuscitation.

CARDIAC TAMPONADE

Cardiac tamponade occurs with pericardial effusion, causing pressure against the heart. It may be a complication of trauma, pericarditis, cardiac surgery, pneumothorax, or heart failure. About 50 ml of fluid norm ally circulates in the pericardial area to reduce friction, and a sudden increase in this volume or fluid or leaking of air from a pneumothorax into the pericardial sac can compress the heart, causing a number of cardiac responses:

- Increased end-diastolic pressure in both ventricles.
- Decrease in venous return.
- Decrease in ventricular filling.

Symptoms may include pressure or pain in the chest, dyspnea, and pulsus paradoxus >10 mm Hg. Beck's triad (increased CVP, distended neck veins, muffled heart sounds, and hypotension) is common. As fluid and clots accumulate in the pericardial sac, they prevent the blood from filling the ventricles and decreases cardiac output and perfusion of the body, including the kidneys (resulting in decreased urinary output). X-rays may show change in cardiac silhouette and mediastinal shift (in 20%). Treatment includes pericardiocentesis with large bore needle or surgical repair to control bleeding and relieve cardiac compression.

HYPOVOLEMIC SHOCK/VOLUME DEFICIT

Hypovolemic shock occurs when there is inadequate intravascular fluid. The loss may be *absolute* because of an internal shifting of fluid, or an external loss of fluid, as occurs with massive hemorrhage, thermal injuries, severe vomiting or diarrhea, and internal injuries (such as ruptured spleen or dissecting arteries) that interfere with intravascular integrity. Hypovolemia may also be *relative* and related to vasodilation, increased capillary membrane permeability from sepsis or injuries, and decreased colloidal osmotic pressure that may occur with loss of sodium and some disorders, such as hypopituitarism and cirrhosis.

Hypovolemic shock is classified according to the degree of fluid loss:

- *Class I:* <750 ml or ≤15% of total circulating volume (TCV).
- *Class II:* 750-1500 ml or 15-30% of TCV.
- *Class III:* 1500-2000 ml or 30-40% of TCV.
- *Class IV:* >2000 ml or >40% of TCV.

SYMPTOMS AND TREATMENT

Hypovolemic shock occurs when the total circulating volume of fluid decreases, leading to a fall in venous return that in turn causes a decrease in ventricular filling and preload, indicated by ↓ in right atrial pressure (RAP) and pulmonary artery occlusion pressure (PAOP). This results in a decrease in stroke volume and cardiac output. This in turn causes generalized arterial vasoconstriction, increasing afterload (↑ systemic vascular resistance), causing decreased tissue perfusion.

Symptoms: anxiety, pallor, cool and clammy skin, delayed capillary refill, cyanosis, hypotension, increasing respirations, weak, thready pulse.

Treatment:

- Treatment is aimed at identifying and treating the cause.
- Administration of blood, blood products, autotransfusion, colloids (such as plasma protein fraction), and/or crystalloids (such as normal saline).
- Oxygen; intubation and ventilation may be necessary.
- Medications may include vasopressors, such as dopamine.

NOTE: Fluids must be given before starting vasopressors!

ANAPHYLAXIS SHOCK

Anaphylactic reaction or anaphylactic shock may present with a few symptoms or a wide range of potentially lethal effects.

Symptoms:

Symptoms may recur after the initial treatment (biphasic anaphylaxis), so careful monitoring is essential:

- Sudden onset of weakness, dizziness, confusion.
- Severe generalized edema and angioedema. Lips and tongue may swell.
- Urticaria
- Increased permeability of vascular system and loss of vascular tone – leading to severe hypotension & shock.
- Laryngospasm/bronchospasm with obstruction of airway causing dyspnea and wheezing.
- Nausea, vomiting, and diarrhea.
- Seizures, coma and death.

Treatments:

- Establish patent airway and intubate if necessary for ventilation.
- Provide oxygen at 100% high flow.
- Monitor VS.
- Administer epinephrine (Epi-pen® or solution).
- Albuterol per nebulizer for bronchospasm.
- Intravenous fluids to provide bolus of fluids for hypotension.
- Diphenhydramine if shock persists.
- Methylprednisolone if no response to other drugs.

BACTEREMIA, SEPTICEMIA, AND SIRS

There are a number of terms used to refer to **severe infections** and often used interchangeably, but they are part of a continuum:

- **Bacteremia** is the presence of bacteria in the blood but without systemic infection.
- **Septicemia** is a systemic infection caused by pathogens (usually bacteria or fungi) present in the blood.
- **Systemic inflammatory response syndrome** (SIRS), a generalized inflammatory response affecting many organ systems, may be caused by infectious or non-infectious agents, such as trauma, burns, adrenal insufficiency, pulmonary embolism, and drug overdose. If an infectious agent is identified or suspected, SIRS is an aspect of sepsis. Infective agents include a wide range of bacteria and fungi, including *Streptococcus pneumoniae* and *Staphylococcus aureus*. **SIRS** includes 2 of the following:
  - Elevated (>38°C) or subnormal rectal temperature (<36°C).
  - Tachypnea or $PaCO_2$ <32 mm Hg.
  - Tachycardia.
  - Leukocytosis (>12,000) or leukopenia (<4000).

SEPSIS, SEVERE SEPSIS, SEPTIC SHOCK, AND MODS

Infections can progress from bacteremia, septicemia, and SIRS to the following:

- **Sepsis** is presence of infection either locally or systemically in which there is a generalized life-threatening inflammatory response (SIRS). It includes all the indications for SIRS as well as one of the following:
  - Changes in mental status.
  - Hypoxemia without preexisting pulmonary disease.
  - Elevation in plasma lactate.
  - Decreased urinary output <5 mL/kg/hr for ≥1 hour.
- **Severe sepsis** includes both indications of SIRS and sepsis as well as indications of increasing organ dysfunction with inadequate perfusion and/or hypotension.
- **Septic shock** is a progression from severe sepsis in which refractory hypotension occurs despite treatment. There may be indications of lactic acidosis.

Multi-organ dysfunction syndrome (MODS) is the most common cause of sepsis-related death. Cardiac function becomes depressed, acute respiratory distress syndrome (ARDS) may develop, and renal failure may follow acute tubular necrosis or cortical necrosis. Thrombocytopenia appears in about 30% of those affected and may result in disseminated intravascular coagulation (DIC). Liver damage and bowel necrosis may occur.

MULTIPLE-ORGAN FAILURE SYNDROME IN POST-SHOCK SETTING

The **multiple-organ failure syndrome** is defined as failure of 2 or more organ systems. The syndrome is recognized in patients who have been revived from the shock state, and occurs as a result of the body's natural systemic response to shock. Typically within 2 to 3 days of resuscitation, the systemic response is initiated; the degree of this response (largely inflammatory in nature) is dependent on the severity of the initial injury caused by the shock state. Although this inflammatory response typically resolves on its own within 2 weeks, in some patients a sustained elevated inflammation may be noted. The persistent inflammatory response results in a continued increase in cell production, which leads to a hypermetabolic, acidotic state, and results in the progressive failure of the organs.

Continuum of Care for Trauma

Patient Safety and Transfer

ASSESSMENT AND PREVENTION OF FALLS

Falls are extremely common in the elderly population and are a significant cause of physical and psychological injury. Risk factors for falls include age over 75, living alone, history of a previous fall, need for a cane or walker, and cognitive, visual or neurological impairment. Elderly patients should be questioned about falls at each visit. An important part of the history is an assessment of the living situation and potential hazards that may exist there. Patients should also be questioned about medications they are taking. Medications that can increase a patient's risk for falling include any drug that is sedating, cardiac and antihypertensive medications, and hypoglycemic drugs. A patient with a history of falling should have a detailed physical exam. Special attention should be given to orthostatic vital signs, joints, and neurological exam, including visual, hearing and nutritional status. The goals of intervention are aimed at reducing the risk of falling. Interventions include education, minimizing risk factors, correcting any underlying cause, and reducing hazards in the home.

PHYSICAL RESTRAINTS

Restraints are used to restrict movement and activity when other methods of controlling patient behavior have failed and there is risk of harm to the patient/others. There are **two primary types of restraints**: violent (behavioral) and non-violent (clinical). Violent restraints are more commonly used in the psychiatric unit or when individuals exhibit aggressive behavior. More commonly, non-violent restraints are used to ensure that the individual does not interfere with safe care. Non-violent restraints are commonly used in the confused elderly or intubated patient to prevent pulling out lines/removing equipment. The federal government and the Joint Commission have issued strict guidelines for temporary restraints or those not part of standard care (such as post-surgical restraint):

- Each facility must have a written policy & restraints are only used when ordered by a physician (usually require written/signed order every 24hrs and within 4 hours of restraint initiation).
- An assessment must be completed frequently, including circulation, toileting, and nutritional needs (generally every 1-2 hours).
- All alternative methods should be tried before applying a restraint & the least restrictive effective restraint should be used.
- A nurse must remove the restraint, assess, and document findings at least every 2 hours; every hour for violent restraints.

Key: Least restrictive option for the least amount of time.

CHEMICAL RESTRAINTS

Chemical restraints involve the use of pharmacological sedatives to manage an individual's behavior problems. This type of restraint is indicated only when severe agitation/violence put the patient at risk for injury to themselves or others. Chemical restraints inhibit the individuals' physical movements, making their behavior more manageable. It is important to realize that medication used on an ongoing basis as part of treatment is not legally considered a chemical restraint, even though the medications may be the same. There is little consensus about the use of chemical restraints, although benzodiazepines and antipsychotics are frequently used to control severe agitation (haloperidol, lorazepam, etc.). Oral medications should be tried first before injections, as oral medication is less coercive. It is important for the nurse to realize that chemical restraints are used as a last resort when other measures (such as de-

55

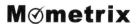

escalation and environmental modification) have failed and there is an immediate risk of harm to the patient or others.

PREVENTING ADDITIONAL INJURY TO TRAUMA PATIENT UPON ARRIVAL TO TRAUMA UNIT

Methods for **preventing additional injury** to the trauma patient upon arrival to the trauma unit include:

- **Supervision**: Someone should stay with the patient until the patient is stabilized enough to be safely left unattended. This is especially important if the patient is unconscious at the time of admission, confused, or disoriented.
- **Safety measures:** Patients should have siderails and safety straps to prevent falls. The call light should be placed by the patient's hand for ease of use and the patient instructed how to use.
- **Padding**: Patients who are thrashing about or restless should have side rails padded so that they don't inadvertently injure themselves.
- **Analgesia**: Pain may cause a patient to thrash about or try to climb of a stretcher, resulting in a fall or dislodging IV's, so the patient should receive adequate medication to relieve pain.
- **Information**: The patient and/or family should be kept informed about interventions and plan of care.

NOSOCOMIAL INFECTION

A **nosocomial infection** is an infection that a patient develops during his or her hospital stay; it also may be called a hospital-acquired infection, or a health care–associated infection. For an infection to be considered nosocomial, it must occur 48 hours or more after the patient is admitted to the hospital, to be sure that the patient was not infected prior to admission. An infection may also be considered nosocomial if it develops within 30 days of the patient's discharge from the hospital. Some infections, when introduced to a patient, can spread like wildfire from one patient to another if proper precautions are not taken.

MODES OF TRANSMISSION

There are 6 known **routes of microorganism transmission** involved in the spread of infection.

- The first mode is **direct-contact transmission**, in which an organism is transferred from an infected individual to a susceptible individual through direct bodily contact.
- **Indirect-contact transmission** occurs when an infected individual touches and contaminates an object (phone, sink, glove), and the object transmits the organism to another individual.
- **Common vehicle transmission** is similar to indirect-contact transmission, but the organism is transmitted through food, water, or medication.
- When an infected individual coughs or sneezes, organism-containing droplets can land on another individual, resulting in **droplet transmission**.
- **Airborne transmission** is similar, except that the organisms within the droplets can remain suspended in the air for long periods of time and be inhaled by another individual.
- A less common mode of transmission in hospitals is **vector-borne transmission,** in which organisms are transferred to the individual through a carrier such as a mosquito.

REDUCING SPREAD OF INFECTION AMONG PATIENTS

Perhaps the most important guidelines for the **prevention of transmission** between both patients and health care workers are the Universal Precautions guidelines, which state that every patient should be regarded as potentially infectious with regard to handling anything that could potentially transmit a bloodborne pathogen (such as the HIV virus or hepatitis C virus). This includes the handling of blood, tissue, semen, vaginal secretions, and body cavity fluids (synovial, cerebrospinal, pleural, pericardial, peritoneal, and amniotic). Treating every patient as potentially infectious ensures that the most care is

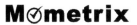

taken to protect all patients. This includes wearing gloves (and changing them between patients), gowns, and other protection as necessary. Disposable items should be used whenever possible, and items that cannot be discarded must be disinfected. Frequent and proper hand washing is also extremely important, and all health care workers should keep nails short and clean, as bacteria can hide under long nails and be transferred to patients.

BENEFITS OF INTERDISCIPLINARY TEAM APPROACH

The **interdisciplinary team** approach to care coordination is beneficial to the patient in several ways. First, the quality of patient care is improved because several different medical services are involved in the care of the patient, and each service is familiar with the patient's situation as a result of increased communication with other health care workers. The interdisciplinary team approach also allows the patient to have a more active role in his or her care because of the emphasis on communication between the patient and all the team members. When the clinicians work together, they also make better use of time spent with the patient, so that the patient is not subjected to lengthy history-taking sessions and redundant testing by unaware clinicians.

ELEMENTS OF CARE PROVIDED PRIOR TO PATIENT ARRIVAL TO A TRAUMA CENTER

Elements of **care provided in the field prior** to patient arrival to a trauma center may include:

- History of injury or illness and mechanism of injury.
- Assessment of airway and provision of oxygen, supraglottic airway device, BVM and/or endotracheal intubation and ventilation.
- Cardiopulmonary resuscitation, including emergency defibrillation.
- ECG and cardiac monitoring, BP monitoring.
- IV line placed and fluid resuscitation begun with target of palpable systolic blood pressure of 70 mm Hg with penetrating trauma and 90 to 110 mm Hg with blunt.
- Control of bleeding with pressure dressings, application of hemostatic gauze, and application of tourniquets.
- Retrieval of amputated body parts and appropriate transport.
- Splinting of fractures, strains, and dislocations; application of cervical collar.
- Immobilization for suspected spinal cord injuries.
- Assessment of level of consciousness, mental status, and neurological status.
- Administration of poison or medication antidotes, such as naloxone for opioid overdose.
- Administration of analgesic medications.
- General assessment of condition, including color and temperature of skin, capillary refill time, tracheal deviation, abnormal respirations, or any other abnormal indications.

CONTINUUM OF CARE

The **continuum of care** refers to a series of services provided for patients or adults needing assistance across a span of time or through stages of change. The continuum of care may involve care practices used from the home, in the community, in a residential care facility, or another institution that provides care. This continuum meets the needs of the adult through stages of health or disability. By having a continuum of care, providers can better identify the needs of patients to provide and coordinate services as needed. For example, if a person needs to move from his home to a long-term care facility for residential treatment because of declining health, the continuum of care can give providers resources for helping the patient to make the transition. The care continuum ensures that all of the client's needs are met while making the transition. The process is tracked and evaluated to ensure competency and that services are complete.

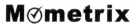

Types and Levels of Service Across Continuum of Care

The continuum of care is a series of care levels that meet patients where they are in terms of health. By identifying the level of the patient's needs, the continuum can guide clinicians for services. On one end is home care and intervention. This provides care for the patient in his home and identifies any additional needs. The next level might be outpatient services, in which the patient receives services at a healthcare center but remains living at home. Beyond this level, the patient may need hospitalization or short-term care. This is more of an acute stage, but the patient does not need services for long. Following this, the patient might need inpatient care or assisted living services, including being monitored on a regular basis and no longer living at home. Finally, the end of the continuum involves high-need care, in which the patient requires intensive treatments because of a fragile state of health.

Forensics

Collecting and Preserving Evidence for Forensic Purposes

Because trauma patients are often transported rapidly to a trauma center, the trauma nurse may be the first person to take steps to **preserve forensic evidence**. In the case of gunshot and stab wounds (which require police reports) or assaults, the trauma nurse should avoid cutting through bullet or stab holes in garments and should place such garments in a plastic or paper bag. All injuries should be carefully described and documented, including the size, number, splatter pattern, and location. If photography is allowed, then photos should be taken before wounds are cleansed and dressed when possible. With gunshot wounds, entry and exit wounds should be noted and counted to determine if a bullet did not exit. If the patient is suspected of firing a gun, then paper bags should be placed over the hands and taped about the wrists so the hands can be tested for gunshot residue. The chain of command protocols should be followed for all evidence.

Chain of Custody of Forensic Evidence Collected from Trauma Patient

Chain-of-custom specimens/items are those for which a facility (such as a laboratory or trauma center) has established a documented record that shows every consecutive person in contact with the specimen/item from the time of collection through transfer and to the time of disposition (both internal and external contact and including date, time, and signature) and ensures that no tampering with the specimen has occurred in order to meet legal requirements. The document must outline provisions for securing long-term storage. Chain-of-custom laboratory specimens may include specimens for blood alcohol, drugs, or crime scene testing, often including blood, urine and DNA testing. The chain-of-custom SOP may include labeling requirements, temperature requirements, expected timeline, packing, and transporting specifications. The person from whom the sample is obtained must be clearly identified as well as the name of the collector and the time, date, and location of obtaining the sample. Containers in which a sample is transported should be secured with custody tape.

End-of-Life Issues

Nursing Role in End of Life Care

End of life care encompasses many dimensions. In the trauma setting, nursing staff caring for the dying patient must shift their priorities from life-saving interventions to providing comfort through the management of symptoms and addressing issues unique to the end of life. Nursing care of the dying patient includes providing supportive care and symptom management to ensure patient comfort and prevention of pain and suffering. Common symptoms occurring at the end of life include pain, dyspnea, anxiety and/or agitation, nausea and vomiting and depression. Additionally, the nurse serves as an advocate to the patient and family, providing education on end of life and supporting them in decision making. Emotional and spiritual support is another dimension of end of life care. The nurse serves to assess the emotional and spiritual needs of the patient and family and helps to coordinate resources to meet those needs. Goals of care are established with the patient and family and communicated to all members of the healthcare team.

ROLE IN ORGAN/TISSUE DONATION FOR POSSIBLE CANDIDATES

The trauma nurse should help to **identify potential organ/tissue donors** and ensure that the local organ procurement organization (OPO) is notified as soon as possible so representatives can assess the patient's suitability. In some cases, the patient may carry a donation card, but often the family members make the decision. The nurse must know the exclusions (viral infections, viral hepatitis, TB, untreated septicemia, extracranial malignancies, prion disease, and IV drug user) and the steps needed for brain-injured patients and patients who are potential donors after cardiac death to maintain viability of organs. Families are generally approached by OPO representatives or trained staff rather than trauma personnel (while the patient remains on life support) to ask for permission to obtain organs and tissue for donation. If the family agrees to organ/tissue donation, the trauma nurse can help to coordinate maintenance care and the timing of withdrawal of life support as well as providing emotional support to family members.

SUPPORTING FAMILIES OF DYING PATIENTS

Families of **dying patients** often do not receive adequate support from nursing staff that feel unprepared for dealing with families' grief and unsure of how to provide comfort, but families may be in desperate need of this support:

- **Before death:**
  - Stay with the family and sit quietly, allowing them to talk, cry, or interact if they desire.
  - Avoid platitudes, "His suffering will be over soon."
  - Avoid judgmental reactions to what family members say or do and realize that anger, fear, guilt, and irrational behavior are normal responses to acute grief and stress.
  - Show caring by touching the patient and encouraging family to do the same.
  - Note: Touching hands, arms, or shoulders of family members can provide comfort, but follow clues of the family.
  - Provide referrals to support groups if available.

- **Time of death:**
  - Reassure family measures have been taken to ensure the patient's comfort.
  - Express personal feeling of loss, "She was such a sweet woman, and I'll miss her" and allow family to express feelings and memories. Provide information about what is happening during the dying process, explaining death rales, Cheyne-Stokes respirations, etc.
  - Alert family members to imminent death if they are not present. Assist to contact clergy/spiritual advisors.
  - Respect feelings and needs of parents, siblings, and other family.

- **After death:**
  - Encourage parents/family members to stay with the patient as long as they wish to say goodbye.
  - Use the patient's name when talking to the family.
  - Assist family to make arrangements, such as contacting funeral home.
  - If an autopsy is required, discuss with the family and explain timing.
  - If organ donation is to occur, assist the family to make arrangements. Encourage family members to grieve and express emotions.

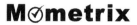

KÜBLER-ROSS'S STAGES OF GRIEF

Grief is a normal response to the death or severe illness/abnormality of a patient. How a person deals with grief is very personal, and each will grieve differently. Elisabeth Kübler-Ross identified **five stages of grief** in *On Death and Dying* (1969), which can apply to both patients and family members. A person may not go through each stage but usually goes through two of the five stages:

- **Denial**: Patients/families may be resistive to information and unable to accept that a person is dying/impaired. They may act stunned, immobile, or detached and may be unable to respond appropriately or remember what's said, often repeatedly asking the same questions.
- **Anger**: As reality becomes clear, patient/families may react with pronounced anger, directed inward or outward. Women, especially, may blame themselves and self-anger may lead to severe depression and guilt, assuming they are to blame because of some personal action. Outward anger, more common in men, may be expressed as overt hostility.
- **Bargaining**: This involves if-then thinking (often directed at a deity): "If I go to church every day, then God will prevent this." Patient/family may change doctors, trying to change the outcome.
- **Depression**: As the patient and family begin to accept the loss, they may become depressed, feeling no one understands and overwhelmed with sadness. They may be tearful or crying and may withdraw or ask to be left alone.
- **Acceptance**: This final stage represents a form of resolution and often occurs outside of the medical environment after months. Patients are able to accept death/dying/incapacity. Families are able to resume their normal activities and lose the constant preoccupation with their loved one. They are able to think of the person without severe pain.

> **Review Video: The Five Stages of Grief**
> Visit mometrix.com/academy and enter code: 648794

HOSPICE CARE

The name hospice is derived from the word hospitality. **Hospice care** is based on the philosophy of the acceptance of the death. The goal of hospice care is to provide a pain-free, dignified setting in which patients can spend their final days. Hospice care is generally recommended when a patient has less than six months to live and conventional treatments have either been exhausted or are considered inappropriate. Hospice care is available in many different settings, including the home, hospital and extended care facilities. Hospice care is generally accomplished by a multidisciplinary team including physicians, nurses, therapists, social workers and clergy. Regular meetings with the team and the family are critical to the success of hospice care.

ADVANCE DIRECTIVES

In accordance to Federal and state laws, individuals have the right to self-determination in health care, including decisions about end of life care through **advance directives** such as **living wills** and the right to assign a surrogate person to make decisions through a **durable power of attorney**. Patients should routinely be questioned about an advanced directive as they may present at a healthcare provider without the document. Patients who have indicated they desire a **do-not-resuscitate (DNR)** order should not receive resuscitative treatments for terminal illness or conditions in which meaningful recovery cannot occur. Patients and families of those with terminal illnesses should be questioned as to whether the patients are hospice patients. For those with DNR requests or those withdrawing life support, staff should provide the patient palliative rather than curative measures, such as pain control and/or oxygen, and emotional support to the patient and family. Religious traditions and beliefs about death should be treated with respect.

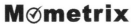

Discharge Planning

Discharge planning begins as soon as a patient is admitted to hospital. The health care team starts educating the patient right away about what to expect and what milestones need to be met before discharge. They also interview the patient about what they want to see happen upon discharge. A patient may have had many admissions and will know from the beginning that they can no longer handle self-care at home. The interdisciplinary team would take this information into account when developing a plan of care for this hospitalization and start making contacts with facilities that may be able to handle the patient upon discharge. Discharge planning must be started early to shorten the length of the hospital stay and plan appropriate post-hospital care. These issues are interconnected, everyone should help with the coordination of and communication between all providers and payers.

TRANSITIONAL CARE PLANNING VS. DISCHARGE CARE PLANNING

Transitional care planning is a general term that describes any focused planning for a patient moving through the health care system. It is an all-encompassing term that describes the entire care process, from admission to discharge. There are laws regarding transitional planning that are enforced by legislation. They guide the case manager, and have written performance standards that allow the case manager to meet accreditation standards in the form of policies and procedures. Discharge planning is also mandated by federal law, and is part of transitional care planning. Transitional care planning includes working with other providers and professionals to meet the patient's needs and negotiate with the payer for reimbursement

PURPOSE AND GOALS

Discharge planning is a formal process that allows care providers to coordinate the individual needs of the patient extending beyond their time in a hospital or long-term-care setting. This assessment process examines how to provide the appropriate provider care once they no longer meet criteria for hospitalization. Also considered is an understanding of the patient's insurance and benefit coverage to ensure that needed services will be available without unreasonable financial burden. The patient must receive clear and accurate teaching about their condition and self-care as well as community resources that will be available to them.

Professional Issues

Trauma Quality Management

STEPS TO EVIDENCE-BASED PRACTICE GUIDELINES

Steps to **evidence-based practice guidelines** include:

1. **Focus on the topic/methodology:** This includes outlining possible interventions/treatments for review, choosing patient populations and settings and determining significant outcomes. Search boundaries (such as types of journals, types of studies, dates of studies) should be determined.
2. **Evidence review:** This includes review of literature, critical analysis of studies, and summarizing of results, including pooled meta-analysis.
3. **Expert judgment:** Recommendations based on personal experience from a number of experts may be utilized, especially if there is inadequate evidence based on review, but this subjective evidence should be explicated acknowledged.
4. **Policy considerations:** This includes cost-effectiveness, access to care, insurance coverage, availability of qualified staff, and legal implications.
5. **Policy:** A written policy must be completed with recommendations. Common practice is to utilize letter guidelines, with "A" the most highly recommended, usually based the quality of supporting evidence.
6. **Review:** The completed policy should be submitted to peers for review and comments before instituting the policy.

DEVELOPMENT OF CLINICAL/CRITICAL PATHWAYS

Clinical/critical pathway development is done by those involved in direct patient care. The pathway should require no additional staffing and cover the entire scope of an illness. Steps include:

1. Selection of patient group and diagnosis, procedures, or conditions, based on analysis of data and observations of wide variance in approach to treatment and prioritizing organization and patient needs.
2. Creation of interdisciplinary team of those involved in the process of care, including physicians to develop pathway.
3. Analysis of data includes literature review and study of best practices to identify opportunities for quality improvement.
4. Identification of all categories of care, such as nutrition, medications, nursing.
5. Discussion, reaching consensus.
6. Identifying the levels of care and number of days to be covered by the pathway.
7. Pilot testing and redesigning steps as indicated.
8. Educating staff about standards.
9. Monitoring and tracking variances in order to improve pathways.

LEVELS OF STRENGTH OF EVIDENCE-BASED PRACTICE

LEVELS OF STRENGTH OF EVIDENCE-BASED PRACTICE:

- Level I (A–D) – Meta-analysis or a number of controlled studies together.
- Level II (A–D) – Individual experimental study.
- Level III (A–D) – Quasi-experimental study.
- Level IV (A–D) – Nonexperimental study.

- Level V (A–D) – Case report or methodically acquired; confirmable quality or program assessment information.
- Level VI – Judgment of esteemed authorities; also regulatory or legal opinions.

OUTCOMES EVALUATION

Outcomes evaluation is an important component of evidence-based practice, which involves both internal and external research. All treatments are subjected to review to determine if they produce positive outcomes, and policies and protocols for outcomes evaluation should be in place. Outcomes evaluation includes the following:

- **Monitoring** over the course of treatment involves careful observation and record keeping that notes progress, with supporting laboratory and radiographic evidence as indicated by condition and treatment.
- **Evaluating** results includes reviewing records as well as current research to determine if outcomes are within acceptable parameters.
- **Sustaining** involves discontinuing treatment, but continuing to monitor and evaluate.
- **Improving** means to continue the treatment but with additions or modifications in order to improve outcomes.
- **Replacing** the treatment with a different treatment must be done if outcomes evaluation indicates that current treatment is ineffective.

THEORY-PRACTICE GAP

BRIDGING THE GAP

The **theory-practice gap** exists because clinicians and researchers traditionally work in 2 separate worlds; the clinical community is directly involved in patient care on a daily basis, while the research community is removed from the realm of patient care. Both communities, however, have the same goal, and that is to improve patient care and quality of life. Establishing communication and camaraderie between the 2 communities is incredibly beneficial for both sides. Training sessions in which clinicians are educated about research practices and researchers are trained about clinical practices are a good start. Facilitating research collaborations between researchers and clinicians is another great way to improve communication. Clinician-researchers can function as intermediaries between the 2 communities, and can educate others. The development of standard operating procedures or best practice guidelines for the transfer of knowledge is also important.

RESOURCE-BASED VIEW

The **Resource-Based View (RBV)** is a theory first developed by economists with the purpose of determining the resources available to a firm or institution. It is an organizational study of the effectiveness of an institution as a result of the resources available to the institution. When applied to the theory-practice gap, the RBV is that the transfer of knowledge within and between organizations or institutions (in this case, between the clinical setting and the research setting) is costly and difficult, based on the fact that the capacity of the clinical community to absorb knowledge is low. To correct for this, the RBV states that available resources should be used to enhance and expand the learning and absorptive capacity of the clinical community.

INSTITUTIONAL THEORY

Institutional Theory (IT), generally defined, is a theory based on the idea that it is difficult to develop institution-wide rules because there are individuals within the institution to whom the rules may not apply. These generalized institutional rules may not be feasible when applied to the daily practice of the individuals operating within the institution. This results in a gap between the actual rules of the

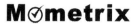

organization and what is done by the individuals within. If the rules are not feasible, the individual may engage in evidence-based decision making. This gap between the rules and the shift to evidence-based decision making will make it more difficult to transfer knowledge both within the clinical community and between the research community and the clinical community.

CRITICAL READING OF RESEARCH ARTICLES

There are a number of steps to **critical reading** to evaluate research:

1. **Consider the source** of the material. If it is in the popular press, it may have little validity compared to something published in a peer-reviewed journal.
2. **Review the author's credentials** to determine if a person is an expert in the field of study.
3. **Determine thesis**, or the central claim of the research. It should be clearly stated.
4. **Examine the organization** of the article, whether it is based on a particular theory, and the type of methodology used.
5. **Review the evidence** to determine how it is used to support the main points. Look for statistical evidence and sample size to determine if the findings have wide applicability.
6. **Evaluate** the overall article to determine if the information seems credible and useful and should be communicated to administration and/or staff.

INTERNAL AND EXTERNAL VALIDITY, GENERALIZABILITY, AND REPLICATION

Many research studies are most concerned with **internal validity** (adequate unbiased data properly collected and analyzed within the population studied), but studies that determine the efficacy of procedures or treatments, for example, should have **external validity** as well; that is, the results should be **generalizable** (true) for similar populations. **Replication** of the study with different subjects, researchers, and under different circumstances should produce similar results. For various reasons, some people may be excluded from a study so that instead of randomized subjects, the subjects may be highly selected so when data is compared with another population in which there is less or more selection, results may be different. The selection of subjects, in this case, would interfere with external validity. Part of the design of a study should include considerations of whether or not it should have external validity or whether there is value for the institution based solely on internal validation.

SELECTION AND INFORMATION BIAS

Selection bias occurs when the method of selecting subjects results in a cohort that is not representative of the target population because of inherent error in design. For example, if all patients who develop urinary infections are evaluated per urine culture and sensitivities for microbial resistance, but only those patients with clinically-evident infections are included, a number of patients with sub-clinical infections may be missed, skewing the results. Selection bias is only a concern when participants in studies are specifically chosen. Many surveillance studies do not involve selection of subjects.

Information bias occurs when there are errors in classification, so an estimate of association is incorrect. Non-differential misclassification occurs when there is similar misclassification of disease or exposure among both those who are diseased/exposed and those who are not. Differential misclassification occurs when there is a differing misclassification of disease or exposure among both those who are diseased/exposed and those who are not.

Qualitative and Quantitative Data

Both **qualitative and quantitative data** are used for analysis, but the focus is quite different:

- **Qualitative data**: Data are described verbally or graphically, and the results are subjective, depending upon observers to provide information. Interviews may be used as a tool to gather information, and the researcher's interpretation of data is important. Gathering this type of data can be time-intensive, and it can usually not be generalized to a larger population. This type of information gathering is often useful at the beginning of the design process for data collection.
- **Quantitative data**: Data are described in terms of numbers within a statistical format. This type of information gathering is done after the design of data collection is outlined, usually in later stages. Tools may include surveys, questionnaires, or other methods of obtaining numerical data. The researcher's role is objective.

Hypothesis

A **hypothesis** should be generated about the probable cause of the disease/infection based on the information available in laboratory and medical records, epidemiologic study, literature review, and expert opinion. A hypothesis, for example, should include the infective agent, the likely source, and the mode of transmission: "Wound infections with *Staphylococcus aureus* were caused by reuse and inadequate sterilization of single-use irrigation syringes used during wound care in the ICU."

Hypothesis Testing

Hypothesis testing includes data analysis, laboratory findings, and outcomes of environmental testing. It usually includes case control studies, with 2-4 controls picked for each case of infection. They may be matched according to age, sex, or other characteristics, but they are not infected at the time they are picked for the study. Cohort studies, whose controls are picked based on having or lacking exposure, may also be instituted. If the hypothesis cannot be supported, then a new hypothesis or different testing methods may be necessary.

Research Resources Available to Clinicians

Nurses, nurse practitioners, physicians, and other clinicians are often too busy to devote time to exploring the latest research advances, which could potentially be used to institute a change in practice that would greatly benefit patients. Reviewing literature can be a tedious and time-consuming process that just does not fit into the schedule of the busy clinician. There are ways that clinicians can find information about the latest practice changes and new guidelines; organizations like the Centers for Disease Control and Prevention (CDC), the National Institutes of Health (NIH), the National Cancer Institute (NCI), and the AACN often provide this information. These organizations review the literature and develop best practices, research-based protocols, and guidelines for clinicians to follow when instituting practice changes.

Outcomes Management

Outcomes management is defined by Wojner as "the enhancement of physiologic and psychosocial patient outcomes through development and implementation of exemplary health practices and services, as driven by outcomes assessment." An alternate definition of outcomes management, as stated by Ellwood, is "a technology of patient experience designed to help patients, payers, and providers make rational medical care-related choices based on better insight into the effects of these choices on the patient's life." Although the two men had different definitions for outcome management, the line of thinking is the same, and that is the importance of a link between patient outcomes and quality control measures used to ensure that the best possible outcomes are arrived at as often as possible.

APPLICATION OF QUALITY IMPROVEMENT PROCESSES AND PRACTICES

Steps to take when applying **quality improvement processes and practice** include:

1. Build relationships among staff in order to facilitate change.
2. Assess needs of the organizations, the climate for change, and the extent of support and resistance in the organization.
3. Produce an internal action plan that describes problems that need resolution, development needs, and process steps to be completed, outlining responsible staff and a timeline for completion of tasks.
4. Delineate resource needs, including staffing and training, with a detailed budget outlining the statistical, clerical, and technical needs.
5. Clarify roles and responsibilities organization-wide.
6. Educate regarding the mission, vision, values, philosophy of quality management, techniques and tools, benefits, and accreditation and regulatory needs.

A **cost-benefit analysis** should be conducted, using average cost of an event and the cost of intervention to demonstrate savings. For example, if an institution were averaging 10 surgical site infections annually at a cost of $300,000 and if intervention costs (including staff, training, and materials) were $126,000, the annual cost benefit would be $174,000.

ACCOMPLISHING QI

Quality improvement (QI) is accomplished through peer review or another form of assessment. In peer review, the approach is to acknowledge and prize the work nurses do. This shows the way toward better standards of work and puts off work that is not within what the nurse can legally do. It heightens the quality of medical attention and gives a means for attaining answerability and conscientiousness. Another form of assessment may include an audit, question/answer or appraisal, or patient contentment question/answer or appraisal.

Risk management – Organizations and actions meant to acknowledge and intercede resulting in less chance of harm to a patient and ensuing claims in opposition to the medical attention workers. This is founded on the supposition that a lot of harm done to patients could be stopped from happening in the first place. Risk management is an assessment of places when legal responsibility is an issue, like patients, methods, or how accounts are maintained. Risk management also involves instruction used to lessen the chance of a problem in a recognized part.

OUTCOMES MANAGEMENT QUALITY MODEL
PHASE 1

The **outcomes management quality model** has 4 separate phases. The **first phase** includes the identification of long-term outcomes for the patient in order to gauge the length of the time of care and to set a starting point. Another part of phase 1 is the selection of instruments to be used for the longitudinal study; in other words, what instruments are going to be used to determine the long-term care outcomes. These instruments typically assess quality of life, functional status, and patient satisfaction. Phase 1 also includes the identification of intermediate outcomes, which may include setbacks in the patient care process. The identification of variances that lead to setbacks in care (such as laboratory errors or physician errors) is also a part of phase 1. The last important part of phase 1 is the creation of a population database.

PHASE 2

Phase 2 of the outcomes management quality model includes the review of both traditional practice and existing literature. The overall purpose or goal of phase 2 of the model is the development of interdisciplinary practice standards. During phase 2, the members of the interdisciplinary team will gather to discuss and negotiate existing and proposed practice standards. The protocols, pathways, and order sets that are designed and formulated during this period are all considered to be "structured care methodologies" (SCMs). These SCMs will be used on the patient cohort population. Once the interdisciplinary team has decided on a set of SCMs for the cohort, the entire initiative can be standardized.

PHASE 3

Phase 3 of the outcomes management quality model is the actual implementation of the structured care methodologies within the patient cohort population. These newly instituted structured care methodologies become the standard of practice, and once the members of the interdisciplinary team and other pertinent staff members are educated about the new practices, data collection can be initiated. If the new practices are expensive (if they require expensive equipment and maintenance, or more supplies, or more billable hours initially), the interdisciplinary team should conduct a cost-benefit analysis, the obvious benefits being that length of stay, number of complications, and number of patient readmissions will be reduced as a result of the new practices.

PHASE 4

Phase 4, the final phase of the outcomes management quality model, involves a thorough, in-depth analysis of the interdisciplinary data that have accumulated during the course of the outcomes management initiative process. Once the data have been analyzed, the interdisciplinary team should meet to discuss whether certain practices or structured care methodologies should be revised to optimize outcomes management. If the team does identify practices that need revision, the initiative will return to phase 2. After this discussion, the interdisciplinary team should discuss any new questions or hypotheses that are related to outcomes management in order to perhaps begin another initiative.

OUTCOME FOLLOW-UP AND FEEDBACK TO EMS TEAM AND REFERRING FACILITIES

Trauma center **outcome follow-up** may vary depending on the type of trauma and patient transfers. Outcome follow-up may include scheduled follow-up visits to assess patient's progress and compliance with treatment. In some cases, telephone follow-up may be carried out at scheduled intervals, such as one week after discharge and at one month and 6 months. Surveys may be sent to patients after discharge by mail or email. If agreements are in place to share electronic health records in compliance with HIPAA regulations, then information about the patient's status may be obtained directly from records. According to the American College of Surgeons Committee on Trauma (ACS-COT), trauma centers must **provide feedback** to referring facilities as well as EMS teams. This feedback may be provided in a similar manner as outcome follow-up, such as through telephone calls, emails, access to electronic health records as well as discharge summaries. Feedback should include information regarding resuscitation, assessment of injuries at time of admission, treatments provided, patient education, information about transfers and/or discharges, and transfusion protocols utilized.

MORTALITY AND MORBIDITY REVIEW

Mortality and morbidity reviews are confidential discussions of sentinel events and serious incidents/complications in order to explore exactly what happened, if standards of care were breached, where errors occurred, what was done correctly, why the event/incident/complication occurred, what steps can be taken to avoid a recurrence of this same type of problems, and what can be learned. The format for the MMR may vary from one organization to another. MMRs may be routinely scheduled or scheduled in response to problems although typically the number of cases should be limited to ≤3 per meeting. Attendance is generally mandatory for those involved as well as residents and faculty. The MMR is typically led by an interdisciplinary team with a designated chair person or leader. The case should be presented in an agreed upon format, such as SBAR. It's important that the process be one of learning and process improvement rather than assigning blame or punishing staff members so that members feel free to carry out an open and honest discussion.

Standard Precautions Protecting Staff from Acquiring Infections from Patients

Standard precautions are utilized to protect staff from all blood and body fluids. Elements include:

- **Hand hygiene**: With plain (not antimicrobial) soap or alcohol-based hand rubs.
- **Personal protective equipment**: May include caps, gowns, gloves, goggles, and face guards to protect from spurting or splashing body fluids. PPE should be easily accessed, and use required and enforced by designated personnel.
- **Sharps injury prevention**: Safe injection protocols should be used and sharps disposal containers easily accessible.
- **Cough etiquette**: Patients, families, and staff should be educated about etiquette and provided masks and tissues as needed. Those who are coughing should be advised to stay at least 3 feet away from others.
- **Private rooms**: Used for those who contaminate the environment (uncontrolled diarrhea, cough, etc.) or are unhygienic. If no private room is available, patients with the same colonizing organism may share a space, or patients should be spaced at least 3 feet apart and separated by privacy curtains.
- **Waste disposal**: Protocols should be in place for proper disposal of contaminated supplies and equipment.

Risks and Prevention Interventions for Workplace Violence on Trauma Unit

According to NIOSH, **workplace violence** includes physical assaults, threats, and verbal abuse. Four types of abuse that may occur in a trauma unit include:

- **Criminal activity**: Violence may occur as the result of robbery, such as for drugs, or other criminal activity, such as gang reprisals.
- **Patient/Client-on-worker**: Patients/Clients may attack staff members because of confusion, disorientation, drug use, alcohol use, mental disease, or sociopathic/violent tendencies.
- **Horizontal violence/Worker-on-worker**: Bullying, intimidation, sexual harassment may be directed from one worker to another.
- **Personal-directed**: Confrontations may occur in the workplace between intimate partners.

Risk factors include lack of adequate security, poor lighting, inadequate staffing, patients/families with history of violence and/or substance abuse, poor workplace design, long wait periods, and high crime rates. Prevention interventions include adequate security (personnel, physical barriers, improved lighting, metal detectors, closed circuit TV), effective management, staff training, analysis of hazards in the workplace, routine review of events to assess for patterns or risks, and employee surveys to help identify concerns.

Disaster Management

Disaster

A **disaster** is an event where many people are exposed to hazards that results in injury, death, and damage to property. There are a number of hazards that have the potential to lead to a disaster situation.

In general, they can be classified as natural, technological, or caused by human conflict. Some specific examples of each are as follows:

- **Natural**: Firestorms, flood, land shift, tornado, epidemic, earthquake, volcano, hurricane, high winds, blizzard, heat wave.
- **Technological**: Hazmat spills, explosions, utility failure, building collapse, transportation accident, power outage, nuclear accident, dam failure, fire, water loss, ruptured gas main.
- **Human Conflict**: Riots, strikes, suicide bombings, bomb threat, employee violence, mass shootings, equipment sabotage, hostage events, transportation disruption, weapons of mass destruction, computer viruses/worms.

STAGES OF DISASTER/EMERGENCY RESPONSE WITHIN WORKPLACE

Once a disaster has occurred in the workplace, there are **five basic stages** of the response process. They are as follows (in order of operation):

- Recognition that a disaster has occurred.
- Notification of management and employees of the disaster.
- Take steps to guarantee the immediate safety of employees.
- Take steps to guarantee public safety, protection of property.
- Protection of the environment.

The length of each stage depends on the scope of the disaster and how well previous stages were executed. Because people are the first priority of any disaster/emergency response, if there are any people left in harm's way, property and the environment cannot become a focus of protection.

TERRORISM

Terrorism is defined as the use of violence (or threat of violence) to frighten and coerce governments or societies into accepting the instigator's (terrorists) demands. The demands and goals of terrorists are often extreme and focused on areas with high population densities. This means that large companies can become potential targets of a terrorist attack. For this reason, when developing an emergency preparedness/disaster management plan, terrorist attacks should be included as a potential disaster. There are many different possible ways that terrorists can strike. Some examples are weapons of mass destruction, biological agents (i.e. bacteria, viruses, or toxins), nuclear and radiological incidents, incendiary devices, chemicals, and explosive devices.

DISASTER RECOVERY

Disaster recovery is the final stage of any disaster response and deals with the actions necessary to return the disaster site to normal. The recovery effort can be divided into two different periods: restoration and reconstruction/replacement. The restoration period is an immediate recovery step in which the area is made safe, utilities repaired, wreckage removed, and evacuees are allowed to return. The reconstruction/replacement period is a longer process where the disaster area is rebuilt and returned to its pre-disaster condition, both physically and economically. The reconstruction period can take many years and is dependent on the degree of damage and availability of resources for reconstruction efforts. As a part of the disaster recovery process, steps should be taken to prevent a recurrence of the disaster in the future.

CISM

Critical incident stress management (CISM) is a procedure to help people cope with stressful events, such as disasters and traumas, in order to reduce incidence of post-traumatic stress syndrome.

- Defusing sessions usually occur very early, sometimes during or immediately after a stressful event, and are used to educate personnel who are actively involved about what to expect over the next few days and to provide guidance in handling feelings and stress.
- Debriefing sessions usually follow in one to three days and may be repeated periodically as needed. These sessions may include people who were directly involved as well as those indirectly involved. People are encouraged to express their feelings and emotions about the event. The six phases of debriefing include introduction, fact sharing, discussing feelings, describing symptoms, teaching, and reentry. Critiquing the event or attempting to place blame is not productive as part of the CISM process.
- Follow-up is done at the end of the process, usually after about week but this can vary.

Regulations and Standards

EMTALA

The ***Emergency Medical Treatment and Active Labor Act*** (EMTALA) is designed to prevent patient "dumping" from emergency departments (ED), including trauma centers, and is an issue of concern for risk management, requiring staff training for compliance:

- Transfers from the ED may be intrahospital or to another facility.
- Stabilization of the patient with emergency conditions or active labor must be done in the ED prior to transfer, and initial screening must be given prior to inquiring about insurance or ability to pay.
- Stabilization requires treatment for emergency conditions and reasonable belief that, although the emergency condition may not be completely resolved, the patient's condition will not deteriorate during transfer.
- Women in the ED in active labor should deliver both the child and placenta before transfer.
- The receiving department or facility should be capable of treating the patient and dealing with complications that might occur.
- Transfer to another facility is indicated if the patient requires specialized services not available intrahospital, such as to burn centers.

TRAUMA CENTER LEVELS

Trauma centers are designated according to state or local legislative criteria regulation and verified by the American College of Surgeons (ACS). The ACS provides voluntary verification (3-year process) according to the resources available at the center, performance, and the numbers of patients served. A center may have different levels for adult and pediatric care. Levels:

- **Level I** (highest): Can provide complete care for all types and every aspect of injuries, including 24-hour general surgeons and various specialists and can provide rehabilitation services, cardiac surgery, hemodialysis, and microsurgery.
- **Level II**: Similar to level I, but less comprehensive and must transfer some patients to level I for tertiary care.
- **Level III**: ED has 24-hour immediate care by physicians and surgeons/anesthesiologists promptly available. Tend to serve rural communities. Not all subspecialties are available, but can transfer patients to level I or II centers.

- **Level IV**: ED with trauma nurse(s) and physician(s) available on patient arrival and can provide advanced life support and stabilization for transfer.
- **Level V** (lowest): Basic ED with trauma nurse(s) and physician(s) available on patient arrival and may provide surgery and critical-care services with transfer agreements to level I-II trauma centers.

PATIENT'S/FAMILY'S RIGHTS AND RESPONSIBILITIES

Empowering patients and families to act as their own advocates requires they have a clear understanding of their **rights and responsibilities.** These should be given (in print form) and/or presented (audio/video) to patients and families on admission or as soon as possible:

- **Rights** should include competent, non-discriminatory medical care that respects privacy and allows participation in decisions about care and the right to refuse care. They should have clear understandable explanations of treatments, options, and conditions, including outcomes. They should be apprised of transfers, changes in care plan, and advance directives. They should have access to medical records information about charges.
- **Responsibilities should include** providing honest and thorough information about health issues and medical history. They should ask for clarification if they don't understand information that is provided to them, and they should follow the plan of care that is outlined or explain why that is not possible. They should treat staff and other patients with respect.

> **Review Video: Patient Advocacy**
> Visit mometrix.com/academy and enter code: 202160

INCORPORATING PATIENT/FAMILY RIGHTS INTO PLAN OF CARE

In order for **patient/family rights** to be incorporated into the plan of care, the care plan needs to be designed as a collaborative effort that encourages participation of patients and family members. There are a number of different programs that can be useful, such as including patients and families on advisory committees. Additionally, assessment tools, such as surveys for patients/families, can be utilized to gain insight in the issues that are important to them. While infants and small children and sometimes the elderly cannot speak for themselves, "patient" is generally understood to include not only the immediate family but also other groups or communities who have an interest in the care of an individual or individuals. Because many hospital stays are now short-term, programs that include follow-up interviews and assessments are especially valuable in determining if the needs of the patient/family were addressed in the care plan.

INFORMED CONSENT

Patients or guardians must provide **informed consent** for all treatment the patient receives. This includes a thorough explanation of all procedures and treatment and associated risks. Patients/guardians should be apprised of all options and allowed input on the type of treatments. Patients/guardians should be apprised of all reasonable risks and any complications that might be life threatening or increase morbidity. The American Medical Association has established **guidelines for informed consent:**

- Explanation of diagnosis.
- Nature of, and reason for, treatment or procedure.
- Risks and benefits.
- Alternative options (regardless of cost or insurance coverage).
- Risks and benefits of alternative options.
- Risks and benefits of not having a treatment or procedure.
- Providing informed consent is a requirement of all states.

Note: A patient may waive their right to informed consent; if this is the case, the nurse should document the patient's refusal and proceed with the procedure. Also, informed consent is not necessary for procedures performed to save a life/limb in which the patient/family is unable to consent.

CONFIDENTIALITY

Confidentiality is the obligation that is present in a professional-patient relationship. Nurses are under an obligation to protect the information they possess concerning the patient and family. Care should be taken to safeguard that information and provide the privacy that the family deserves. This is accomplished through the use of required passwords when family call for information about the patient and through the limitation of who is allowed to visit. There may be times when confidentiality must be broken to save the life of a patient, but those circumstances are rare. The nurse must make all efforts to safeguard patient records and identification. Computerized record keeping should be done in such a way that the screen is not visible to others, and paper records must be secured.

> **Review Video: Ethics and Confidentiality in Counseling**
> Visit mometrix.com/academy and enter code: 250384

HIPAA

HIPAA refers to the **Health Insurance Portability and Accountability Act of 1996,** under Public Law 104-191. This has a goal of better organization and helpfulness in the medical system, which is to be done by regulating the way that electronic communications for administrative and economic information is done. The requirements include particular transaction regulations (including code sets), security and electronic signatures, privacy and particular identifiers that also have utilization permissions for bosses, health plans and people who give medical attention.

PRIVACY PROVISIONS

HIPAA regulations are designed to protect the rights of individuals regarding the privacy of their health information. The nurse must not release any information or documentation about an individual's **condition or treatment** without consent, as the individual has the right to determine who has access to personal information. Personal information about the individual is considered **protected health information** (PHI), and consists of any identifying or personal information about the individual, such as health history, condition, or treatments in any form, and any documentation, including electronic, oral, or written. Personal information can be shared with a spouse, legal guardians, those with durable power of attorney for the individual, and those involved in care of the individual, such as physicians, without a specific release, but the individual should always be consulted if personal information is to be discussed with others present to ensure there is no objection. Failure to comply with HIPAA regulations can result in the nurse and their employer being held liable and assessed heavy penalties.

SENSITIVE INFORMATION

Sensitive information is classified under HIPAA as protected health information (PHI) and includes

- Any information about an individual's past, present, or future health or condition (mental or physical)
- Any information describing health care provided to the individual
- Any information related to payment for healthcare services that can be used to identify the person
- Any identifying information: name, address, Social Security number, birthdate, and any document or material that contains the identifying information (such as laboratory records)

Information that is to be shared or aggregated for research purposes must first be deidentified. The HIPAA privacy rule provides two methods of deidentification:

- Expert determination (based on applying statistical or scientific principles): The expert must have appropriate knowledge and must document the method and analysis results.
- Safe harbor (removing 18 types of identifiers): includes names, geographic information, zip codes, telephone numbers, license numbers, account numbers, fax numbers, serial numbers of devices, email addresses, URLs, full-face photographs, dates (except year) and biometric identifiers

INDIVIDUAL RIGHTS
HIPAA individual rights:

- Covered entity duties and contact name, title, or telephone to take delivery of grievances with effectual month, day, and year.
- Access, with the right to look at and get a copy of PHI in a designated record set (DRS) in an appropriate time frame.
- Amendment, so that each patient has the right for Covered Entity amend PHI, but this can be not approved by Covered Entity even when the account is correct and finished.
- Accounting, so that the patient has the right to get a record of what information was given out from PHI for 6 years (or less) before the month, day and year that it was asked for.
- Asked for restrictions, so that the patient can ask for limitations of utilization and giving out PHI (although Covered Entity may not allow).
- Confidential communication, so that the provider has to allow and accommodate justifiable desires for PHI information that was exchanged by alternative methods and to alternative places.
- Grievances to covered Entity.
- Grievances to Secretary (HHS/OCR).

CMP
Civil Monetary Penalties (CMP) cost $100 for each infringement. The most one would have to pay is $25,000 for one calendar year for every condition or prohibition that is infringed upon. It is a criminal penalty to unlawfully give out information, with these consequences:

- Up to $50,000 plus a year of jail time.
- Up to $100,000 plus 5 years of jail time for information given out with false pretenses.
- Up to $250,000 plus 10 years of jail time for plan to sell, transfer, or utilize the data for commercial reasons, own gain, or malevolent reasons.
- These consequences are maintained by the Department of Justice (DOJ).

TRAUMA REGISTRY
Registries are collections of secondary data about specific patient diagnoses, treatment, procedures, and/or conditions. **Trauma registries** maintain records of severe traumatic injuries, such as those associated with falls, motor vehicle accidents, physical attacks, stabbings, and shootings. All verified level I trauma centers are required by the American College of Surgeons to maintain a trauma registry. Data elements vary but may include specific demographic information, diagnosis, treatment, stages (when appropriate), status codes, abbreviated injury scale (AIS), injury severity scale (ISS), and functional status. A patient is entered into the registry if the patient meets the case definition as defined by the organization. Information for the registry is abstracted from the patient's medical health record. Use of the trauma registry varies, but periodic reports (at least annually) are prepared based on information in the registry, and the data may be used for planning and process improvement. Follow-up of patients in the registry may or may not be carried out.

Education and Outreach

LEARNING STYLES

Not all people are aware of their preferred **learning style**. A range of teaching materials/methods that relates to all 3 learning preferences—visual, auditory, kinesthetic—(and appropriate for different ages) should be available. Part of assessment for teaching involves choosing the right approach based on observation and feedback. Often presenting learners with different options gives a clue to their preferred learning style. Some people have a combined learning style:

- **Visual learners**:Learn best by seeing and reading:
  - Provide written directions, picture guides, or demonstrate procedures. Use charts and diagrams.
  - Provide photos, videos.
- **Auditory learners**:Learn best by listening and talking:
  - Explain procedures while demonstrating and have learner repeat.
  - Plan extra time to discuss and answer questions.
  - Provide audiotapes.
- **Kinesthetic learners:** Learn best by handling, doing, and practicing:
  - Provide hands-on experience throughout teaching.
  - Encourage handling of supplies/equipment.
  - Allow learner to demonstrate.
  - Minimize instructions and allow person to explore equipment and procedures.

PRINCIPLES OF ADULT LEARNING

Adults have a wealth of life and/or employment experiences. Their attitudes toward education may vary considerably. There are, however, some **principles of adult learning** and typical characteristics of adult learners that an instructor should consider when planning strategies for teaching parents, families, or staff:

- **Practical and goal-oriented:**
  - Provide overviews or summaries and examples.
  - Use collaborative discussions with problem-solving exercises.
  - Remain organized with the goal in mind.
- **Self-directed:**
  - Provide active involvement, asking for input.
  - Allow different options toward achieving the goal.
  - Give them responsibilities.
- **Knowledgeable:**
  - Show respect for their life experiences/ education.
  - Validate their knowledge and ask for feedback.
  - Relate new material to information with which they are familiar.
- **Relevancy-oriented:**
  - Explain how information will be applied.
  - Clearly identify objectives.

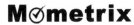

- **Motivated:**
  - o Provide certificates of professional advancement and/or continuing education credit for staff when possible.

BLOOM'S TAXONOMY AND 3 TYPES OF LEARNING

Bloom's taxonomy outlines behaviors that are necessary for learning:

- **Cognitive** - Gaining intellectual skills to master 6 categories of effective learning
  - o Knowledge
  - o Comprehension
  - o Application
  - o Analysis
  - o Synthesis
  - o Evaluation

- **Affective** - Recognizing 5 categories of feelings and values
  - o Receiving phenomena: Accepting need to learn.
  - o Responding to phenomena: Taking active part in care.
  - o Valuing: Understanding value of becoming independent in care.
  - o Organizing values: Understanding how surgery/treatment has improved life.
  - o Internalizing values: Accepting condition as part of life, being consistent and self-reliant.

- **Psychomotor** - Mastering 6 motor skills necessary for independence
  - o Perception: Uses sensory information to learn tasks.
  - o Set: Shows willingness to perform tasks.
  - o Guided response: Follows directions.
  - o Mechanism: Does specific tasks.
  - o Complex overt response: Displays competence in self-care.
  - o Adaptation: Modifies procedures as needed.
  - o Origination: Creatively deals with problems.

LEARNER OUTCOMES

When the quality professional plans an educational offering, whether it be a class, an online module, a workshop, or educational materials, the professional should identify **learner outcomes,** which should be conveyed to the learners from the very beginning so that they are aware of the expectations. The subject matter of the educational material and the learner outcomes should be directly related. For example, if the quality professional is giving a class on decontamination of the environment, then a learner outcome might be: "Identify the difference between disinfectants and antiseptics." There may be one or multiple learner outcomes, but part of the assessment at the end of the learning experience should be to determine if, in fact, the learner outcomes have been achieved. A survey of whether or not the learners felt that they had achieved the learner outcomes can give valuable feedback and guidance to the quality professional.

DEVELOPMENT OF GOALS, MEASURABLE OBJECTIVES, AND LESSON PLANS

Once a topic for performance improvement education has been chosen, then **goals, measurable objectives with strategies, and lesson plans** must be developed. A class should stay focused on one area rather than trying to cover many things. For example:

- **Goal**: Increase compliance with hand hygiene standards in ICU.
- **Objectives:** Develop series of posters and fliers by June 1.
  - o Observe 100% compliance with hand hygiene standards at 2 weeks, 1-month, and 2-month intervals after training is completed.
- **Strategies:** Conduct 4 classes at different times over a one-week period, May 25-31.
  - o Place posters in all nursing units, staff rooms, and utility rooms by January 3.
  - o Develop a slide show presentation for class and Intranet/Internet for access by all staff by May 25.
  - o Utilize handwashing kits.
- **Lesson plans:** Discussion period: Why do we need 100% compliance?
  - o Slide show: The case for hand hygiene.
  - o Discussion: What did you learn?
  - o Demonstration and activities to show effectiveness
  - o Handwashing technique.

APPROACHES TO TEACHING

There are many **approaches to teaching**, and the nurse educator must prepare, present, and coordinate a wide range of educational workshops, lectures, discussions, and one-on-one instructions on any chosen topic. All types of classes will be needed, depending upon the purpose and material:

- **Educational workshops** are usually conducted with small groups, allowing for maximal participation and are especially good for demonstrations and practice sessions.
- **Lectures** are often used for more academic or detailed information that may include questions and answers but limits discussion. An effective lecture should include some audiovisual support.
- **Discussions** are best with small groups so that people can actively participate. This is a good method for problem solving.
- **One-on-one instruction** is especially helpful for targeted instruction in procedures for individuals.
- **Computer/Internet modules** are good for independent learners.

Participants should be asked to evaluate the presentations in the forms of surveys or suggestions, but ultimately the program is evaluated in terms of patient outcomes.

ONE-ON-ONE INSTRUCTION AND GROUP INSTRUCTION FOR PATIENT/FAMILY EDUCATION

Both **one-on-one instruction** and **group instruction** have a place in patient/family education:

- **One-on-one instruction** is the costliest for an institution because it is time intensive. However, it allows the patient and family more interaction with the nurse instructor and allows them to have more control over the process by asking questions or having the instructor repeat explanations or demonstrations. One-on-one instruction is especially valuable when patients and families must learn particular skills, such as managing dialysis, or if confidentiality is important.

- **Group instruction** is the less costly because the needs of a number of people can be met at one time. Group presentations are more planned and usually scheduled for a particular time period (an hour, for example), so patients and families have less control. Questioning is usually more limited and may be done only at the end. Group instruction allows patients/families with similar health problems to interact. Group instruction is especially useful for general types of instruction, such as managing diet or other lifestyle issues.

VIDEOS

Videos are a useful adjunct to teaching as they reduce the time needed for one-on-one instruction (increasing cost-effectiveness). Passive presentation of videos, such as in the waiting area, has little value, but focused viewing in which the nurse discusses the purpose of the video presentation prior to viewing and then is available for discussion after viewing can be very effective. Patients and/or families are often nervous about learning patient care and are unsure of their abilities, so they may not focus completely when the nurse is presenting information. Allowing the patients/families to watch a video demonstration or explanation first and allowing them to stop or review the video presentation can help them to grasp the fundamentals before they have to apply them, relieving some of the anxiety they may be experiencing. Videos are much more effective than written materials for those with low literacy or poor English skills. The nurse should always be available to answer questions and discuss the material after the patients/families finish viewing.

READABILITY

Studies have indicated that learning is more effective if oral presentations and/or demonstrations are supplemented with reading materials, such as handouts. **Readability** (the grade level of material) is a concern because many patients and families may have limited English skills or low literacy, and it can be difficult for the nurse to assess people's reading level. The average American reads effectively at the 6th to 8th grade level (regardless of education achieved), but many health education materials have a much higher readability level. Additionally, research indicates that even people with much higher reading skills learn medical and health information most effectively when the material is presented at the 6th to 8th grade readability level. Therefore, patient education materials (and consent forms) should not be written at higher than 6th to 8th grade level. Readability index calculators are available on the Internet to give an approximation of grade level and difficulty for those preparing materials without expertise in teaching reading.

INSTRUCTING AND ADVISING STAFF ON CHANGES IN POLICIES, PROCEDURES, OR WORKING STANDARDS

Changes in policies, procedures, or working standards are common and the quality professional is responsible for educating the staff about changes related to processes, which should be communicated to staff in an effective and timely manner:

- **Policies** are usually changed after a period of discussion and review by administration and staff, so all staff should be made aware of policies under discussion. Preliminary information should be disseminated to staff regarding the issue during meetings or through printed notices.
- **Procedures** may be changed to increase efficiency or improve patient safety often as the result of surveillance and data about outcomes. Procedural changes are best communicated in workshops with demonstrations. Posters and handouts should be available as well.
- **Working standards** are often changed because of regulatory or accrediting requirements and this information should be covered extensively in a variety of different ways: discussions, workshops, handouts so that the implications are clearly understood.

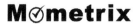

Ethical Issues

ETHICAL ASSESSMENT

While the terms *ethics* and *morals* are sometimes used interchangeably, ethics is a study of morals and encompasses concepts of right and wrong. When making **ethical assessments,** one must consider not only what people should do but also what they actually do, as these two things are sometimes at odds. Ethical issues can be difficult to assess because of personal bias, and that is one of the reasons that sharing concerns with other internal sources and reaching consensus is so valuable. Issues of concern might include options for care, refusal of care, rights to privacy, adequate relief of suffering, and the right to self-determination. Internal sources might include the ethics committee, whose role is to make decisions regarding ethical issues. Risk management can provide guidance related to personal and institutional liability. External agencies might include government agencies, such as the public health department.

BENEFICENCE AND NONMALEFICENCE

Beneficence is an ethical principle that involves performing actions that are for the purpose of benefitting another person. In the care of a patient, any procedure or treatment should be done with the ultimate goal of benefitting the patient, and any actions that are not beneficial should be reconsidered. As conditions change, procedures need to be continually reevaluated to determine if they are still of benefit.

Nonmaleficence is an ethical principle that means healthcare workers should provide care in a manner that does not cause direct intentional harm to the patient:

- The actual act must be good or morally neutral.
- The intent must be only for a good effect.
- A bad effect cannot serve as the means to get to a good effect.
- A good effect must have more benefit than a bad effect has harm.

AUTONOMY AND JUSTICE

Autonomy is the ethical principle that the individual has the right to make decisions about his or her own care. In the case of children or patients with dementia who cannot make autonomous decisions, parents or family members may serve as the legal decision maker. The nurse must keep the patient and/or family fully informed so that they can exercise their autonomy in informed decision-making.

Justice is the ethical principle that relates to the distribution of the limited resources of healthcare benefits to the members of society. These resources must be distributed fairly. This issue may arise if there is only one bed left and two sick patients. Justice comes into play in deciding which patient should stay and which should be transported or otherwise cared for. The decision should be made according to what is best or most just for the patients and not colored by personal bias.

BIOETHICS

Bioethics is a branch of ethics that involves making sure that the medical treatment given is the most morally correct choice given the different options that might be available and the differences inherent in the varied levels of treatment. In the acute/critical care unit, if the patients, family members, and the staff are in agreement when it comes to values and decision-making, then no ethical dilemma exists; however, when there is a difference in value beliefs between the patients/family members and the staff, there is a bioethical dilemma that must be resolved. Sometimes, discussion and explanation can resolve differences, but at times the institution's ethics committee must be brought in to resolve the conflict. The primary goal of bioethics is to determine the most morally correct action using the set of circumstances given.

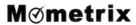

ETHICAL ISSUES RELATED TO TREATMENT OF TERMINALLY ILL PATIENTS

There are a number of ethical concerns that healthcare providers and families must face when determining the treatments that are necessary and appropriate for a terminally-ill patient. It is the nurse's responsibility to provide support and information to help parents/families make informed decisions. Common treatments with their advantages and disadvantages:

- **Analgesia** - Provide comfort. Ease the dying process. Increase sedation and decrease cognition and interaction with family. May hasten death.
- **Active treatments (such as antibiotics, chemotherapy)** - Prolong life. Relieve symptoms. Reassure family. Prolong the dying process. Side effects may be severe (as with chemotherapy).
- **Supplemental nutrition** - Relieve family's anxiety that patient is hungry. Prolong life. May cause nausea, vomiting. May increase tumor growth with cancer. May increase discomfort.
- **IV fluids for hydration** - Relieve family's anxiety that patient is thirsty. Keep mouth moist. May result in congestive heart failure and pulmonary edema with increased dyspnea. Increased urinary output and incontinence may cause skin breakdown. Prolong dying process.
- **Resuscitation efforts** - Allow family to deny death is imminent. Cause unnecessary suffering and prolong dying process.

RESOLVING ETHICAL CONFLICTS

In the health care setting, it is important that **ethical conflicts** be resolved without harming the patient or compromising care. There are several factors that will affect the course and outcome of an ethical conflict.

- First, the level of commitment the clinician has to the patient will determine the amount of effort put forth in resolving an ethical conflict.
- Second, the degree of moral certainty the clinician has will determine the approach to resolution; if the clinician feels that he or she is correct, he or she will most likely not waver in the decision.
- Third, the amount of time available for resolution is important; if the clinician is pressed for time, he or she will most likely come to a decision faster than if there is not a time constraint, in which case avoidance may occur.
- Fourth is the cost-benefit ratio; if the patient refuses to negotiate a certain point, for example, it is not worth the time to the clinician to try to influence the patient's decision.

Testable Tasks

Assessment

HEALTH ASSESSMENT

Health assessment – Gather an account of prior health issues to identify the activities that give the patient more of a chance of problems and can guide instruction for that patient. The health history should include demographics and biographical information. It should include an account of current health problems, including the OPQRST assessment:

- Onset.
- Provocative/palliative (getting well or problem going downhill).
- Quality/quantity.
- Region/radiation.
- Setting.
- Timing.

Discuss prior health issues, including how the patient feels he is generally doing, prior conditions or times in the hospital, harm or operations (including when, what the medical attention was, and what check-ups were done afterwards), emotional well-being, sexual well-being, allergies to food or drugs (and the particular problem that happens including needed medical attention for it if there is any), drugs (prescribed and over-the-counter), immunizations (when and what), sleep routines, and prior assessments for any part of the body. Discuss individual routines, including the utilization of tobacco, alcohol, drugs, caffeine, nutrition, physical activity, hobbies, athletics, and contact sports.

PATIENT HISTORY

A **comprehensive patient history** contains numerous components to help the clinician formulate a diagnosis and treatment plan. Demographic information is an important part of the history, and includes information about the patient's age, sex, and race. The source of the patient referral is also included in the history; it is important to know whether the patient was referred by a primary care physician, a cardiologist, or some other doctor. If someone other than the patient is providing the history, his or her name should be recorded. The chief complaint, or the reason that the patient is being seen, is also important to note, along with a detailed history of the complaint, including when the patient first noticed symptoms, if the symptoms are better or worse at certain times, **and the characteristics of the illness.** Any past medical problems and surgeries are documented as well, including diseases and surgical procedures within the patient's family. Allergies, current medications, and social factors/practices are included in the history.

SCREENING TESTS

When the clinician is asking the patient about his or her past medical history, it is important that the clinician includes questions regarding **screening tests** that the patient may or may not have had recently. If the patient has not had appropriate screening, the clinician should investigate and consider ordering any tests that relate to the patient's current condition. Screening tests such as cholesterol, hemoglobin, and serum glucose are routine blood tests and can be done easily. Urinalysis is another simple screening test, as is a blood pressure reading. More involved and time-consuming tests can be ordered for patients when indicated, including sigmoidoscopy and stool guaiac for routine colon cancer screening, Papanicolaou smear for cervical dysplasia and cancer, mammogram for breast cancer, and ECG for heart abnormalities.

DOCUMENTATION OF FOCUSED HISTORY AND PHYSICAL EXAM

Documentation of a **focused or comprehensive history and physical** exam depends to some degree on the documentation format (SOAP, narrative, PIE, DAR, CBE). Electronic health records may have additional constraints; however, the following elements should be included in documentation:

- **Problems:** The problem list generated, based on patient complaints and assessment, should describe both objective and subjective observations and should be prioritized according to importance (Maslow's hierarchy).
- **Differential diagnoses and nursing diagnoses:** Should be provided for each problem on the list.
- **Further assessment:** Lab tests, screening tests, or imaging that may be needed for items of the problem list should be documented as well as results when they are available.
- **Interventions:** These should be outlined and noted on the plan of care, including any referrals, such as to nutritionist, physical therapist, psychologist/psychiatrist, speech therapist, or occupational therapist.
- **Outcomes:** The results (positive or negative) of interventions should be documented as well as the need for modification.

PHYSICAL HEALTH ASSESSMENT

A **physical health assessment** should include a review of any patient records, a health history, and a general survey of the patient, including the patient's age, general appearance (healthy, unhealthy, hygienic status, mental status, level of consciousness, functional abilities, and obvious abnormalities), height, and weight. The nurse should utilize inspection, palpation, percussion, and auscultation during the examination. The nurse should conduct an organized physical examination. Methods include:

- **Head-to-toe:** This traditional assessment requires examining each part of the body starting with the head and working down through the systems.
- **Functional health patterns (Gordon):** This form of assessment focuses on functional health patterns and includes (1) health perception/management, (2) nutritional/metabolic, (3) elimination, (4) activity/exercise, (5) cognitive/perceptual, (6) sleep/rest, (7) self perception/concept, (8) role/relationship, (9) sexuality/reproductive, (10) coping/stress tolerance, and (11) value/belief.
- **PERSON (basic health needs):** This method, like Gordon's, focuses on functions and includes **P**sychosocial, **E**limination, **R**est/regulatory/reproductive, **S**afety, **O**xygenation, and **N**utrition.

ASSESSMENT TO ESTABLISH MECHANISM OF INJURY

Assessment to establish the **mechanism of injury** includes:

- **Question/Listen:** Reports from the patient (if responsive and cognitively aware), family or friends, and first responders often can establish how an injury occurred, when, and where. Police reports may be available in some cases. The trauma nurse should ask questions to clarify any information provided.
- **Observation:** The patient's general appearance (clean, soiled, unkempt, well-dressed, sporting clothes/uniform), obvious injuries (bruises, swelling, and bleeding), and odor (fruity, alcohol, urine, feces) may provide clues as to the mechanism of injury or the patient's general health and living situation.
- **Physical examination:** The trauma nurse should look for typical patterns of injury associated with different mechanisms of injury. For example, a fall from a height may result in fractures of both feet and back injuries. Hip and wrist fractures are common with falls. Blistering, redness, and sloughing of tissue may suggest burns.

FAST ASSESSMENT

Focused abdominal sonography for trauma (FAST) assessment is a non-invasive ultrasound procedure that is part of the ATLS protocol for assessment of trauma and is generally now used in place of peritoneal lavage to detect free fluid (generally blood). FAST is about 85% to 90% effective in diagnosing intraperitoneal bleeding (usually associated with hepatic or splenic injury) as well as pneumo- and hemothorax (can detect as small a volume as 20 mL, depending on the sonographer's skill), and pericardial effusion associated with blunt or penetrating cardiac trauma. FAST may help to prioritize treatment when a patient presents with multiple penetrating injuries (especially involving inferior chest and superior abdomen). FAST is, however, less effective in identifying bowel injuries. In some cases where patient's condition is not clear, observation and a series of FAST assessments may help to identify problems, such as a slow bleed.

ASSESSMENT OF LOWER EXTREMITIES

Assessment of lower extremities includes a number of different elements:

- **Appearance** includes comparing limbs for obvious differences or changes in skin or nails as well as evaluating for edema, color changes in skin, such as pallor or rubor. Legs that are thin, pale, shiny, and hairless indicate peripheral arterial disease.
- **Perfusion** should be assessed by checking venous filling time and capillary refill, skin temperature (noting changes in one limb or between limbs), bruits (indicating arterial narrowing), pulses (comparing both sides in a proximal to distal progression), ankle-brachial index and toe-brachial index.
- **Sensory function** includes the ability to feel pain, temperature, and touch.
- **Range of motion** of the ankle must be assessed to determine if the joint flexes past 90° because this is necessary for unimpaired walking and aids venous return in the calf.
- **Pain** is an important diagnostic feature of peripheral arterial disease, so the location, intensity, duration, and characteristics of pain are important.

PULSE AND BRUIT

Evaluation of the **pulses** of the lower extremities is an important part of assessment for peripheral arterial disease. Pulses should be first evaluated with the patient in supine position and then again with the legs dependent, checking bilaterally and proximally to distally to determine if intensity of pulse decreases distally. Pedal pulses should be examined at both the posterior tibialis and the dorsalis pedis. The pulse should be evaluated as to the rate, rhythm, and intensity, which is usually graded on a 0-4 scale:

- 0 pulse absent
- 1 weak, difficult to palpate
- 2 normal as expected
- 3 full
- 4 strong and bounding

Pulses may be palpable or absent with peripheral arterial disease. Absence of pulse on both palpation and Doppler probe does indicate peripheral arterial disease.

Bruits may be noted by auscultating over major arteries, such as femoral, popliteal, peroneal, and dorsalis pedis, indicating peripheral arterial disease.

ASSESSMENT OF HEART SOUNDS

Auscultation of **heart sounds** can help to diagnose different cardiac disorders. Areas to auscultate include the aortic area, pulmonic area, Erb's point, tricuspid area, and the apical area. The normal heart sounds represent closing of the valves. The first heart sound (S1) "lub" is closure of the mitral and tricuspid valves (heard at apex/left ventricular area of the heart). The second heart sound (S2) "dub" is closure of the aortic and pulmonic valves (heard at the base of the heart).

Additional Heart Sounds:

- **Gallop rhythms:** *S3* commonly occurs after S2 in children and young adults but may indicate heart failure or left ventricular failure in older adults (heard with patient lying on left side). *S4* occurs before S1, during the contracting of the atria when there is ventricular hypertrophy, found in coronary artery disease, hypertension, or aortic valve stenosis.
- **Opening snap:** Unusual high-pitched sound occurring after S2 with stenosis of mitral valve from rheumatic heart disease.
- **Ejection click:** Brief high-pitched sound after S1; aortic stenosis.
- **Friction rub:** Harsh, grating holosystolic sound; pericarditis.
- **Murmur:** Sound caused by turbulent blood flow from stenotic or malfunctioning valves, congenital defects, or increased blood flow. Murmurs are characterized by location, timing in the cardiac cycle, intensity (rated from Grade I to Grade VI), pitch (low to high-pitched), quality (rumbling, whistling, blowing) and radiation (to the carotids, axilla, neck, shoulder, or back).

ADMINISTRATION OF 12 LEAD ECG

The **electrocardiogram** provides a continuous graphic representation of the electrical activity of the heart. It is indicated for chest pain, dyspnea, syncope, acute coronary syndrome, pulmonary embolism, and possible MI. The standard 12 lead ECG gives a picture of electrical activity from 12 perspectives through placement of 10 body leads:

- 4 limb leads are placed distally on the wrists and ankles (but may be placed more proximally if necessary).
- Precordial leads:
  - V1: right sternal border at 4th intercostal space
  - V2: left sternal border at 4th intercostal space
  - V3: Midway between V2 and V4
  - V4: Left midclavicular line at 5th intercostal space.
  - V5: Horizontal to V4 at left anterior axillary line.
  - V6: Horizontal to V5 at left mid-axillary line.

In some cases, additional leads may be used:

- Right-sided leads are placed on the right in a mirror image of the left leads, usually to diagnose right ventricular infarction through ST elevation.

ELECTROCARDIOGRAM

The **electrocardiogram** records and shows a graphic display of the electrical activity of the heart through a number of different waveforms, complexes, and intervals:

- **P wave**: Start of electrical impulse in the sinus node and spreading through the atria, muscle depolarization.
- **QRS complex:** Ventricular muscle depolarization and atrial repolarization.
- **T wave**: Ventricular muscle repolarization (resting state) as cells regain negative charge.
- **U wave**: Repolarization of the Purkinje fibers.

A modified lead II ECG is often used to monitor basic heart rhythms and dysrhythmias:

- Typical placement of leads for 2-lead ECG is 3 to 5 cm inferior to the right clavicle and left lower ribcage. Typical placement for 3-lead ECG is (RA) right arm near shoulder, (LA) V_5 position over 5th intercostal space, and (LL) left upper leg near groin.

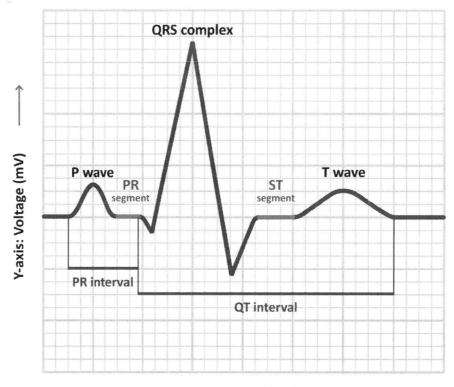

MAP

The **MAP (mean arterial pressure)** is most commonly used to evaluate perfusion as it shows pressure throughout the cardiac cycle. Systole is one-third and diastole two-thirds of the normal cardiac cycle. The MAP for a blood pressure of 120/60 (Normal range 70-100 mm Hg):

$$MAP = \frac{Diastole \times 2 + Systole \times 1}{3}$$

Example: Blood pressure 120/60

$$MAP = \frac{60 \times 2 + 120 \times 1}{3} = \frac{240}{3} = 80$$

JUGULAR VENOUS PRESSURE

Jugular venous pressure (neck-vein) is used to assess the cardiac output and pressure in the right heart as the pulsations relate to changes in pressure in the right atrium. This procedure is usually not accurate if pulse rate is >100. This is a non-invasive estimation of central venous pressure and waveform. Measurement should be done with the internal jugular if possible; if not, the external jugular may be used.

- Elevate the patient's head to 45° (and to 90° if necessary) with patient's head turned to the right.
- Position light at an angle to illuminate veins and shadows.
- Measure the height of the jugular vein pulsation above the sternal joint, using a ruler.
  - Normal height is ≤ 4 cm above sternal angle.
  - Increased pressure (> 4 cm) indicates increased pressure in right atrium and possible right-sided heart failure. It may also indicate pericarditis or tricuspid stenosis. Laughing or coughing may trigger the valsalva response and also cause an increase in pressure.

DIAGNOSTIC PROCEDURES AND TOOLS USED DURING ASSESSMENT OF PULMONARY TRAUMA/DISEASE

The diagnostic procedures and tools used during assessment of **pulmonary and thoracic trauma/disease** will vary according to the type and degree of injury/disease, but may include:

- **Thorough physical examination** including cardiac and pulmonary status, assessing for any abnormalities.
- **Electrocardiogram** to assess for cardiac arrhythmias.
- **Chest x-ray** should be done for all those with injuries to check for fractures, pneumothorax, major injuries, and placement of intubation tubes. X-rays can be taken quickly and with portable equipment so they can be completed quickly during the initial assessment.
- **Computerized tomography** may be indicated after initial assessment, especially if there is a possibility of damage to the parenchyma of the lungs.
- **Oximetry and atrial blood gases** as indicated.
- **12-lead electrocardiogram** may be needed if there are arrhythmias for more careful observation.
- **Echocardiogram** should be done if there is apparent cardiac damage.

KIDNEY REGULATORY FUNCTIONS REGARDING FLUID BALANCE

Kidney regulatory functions include maintaining **fluid balance**. Fluid excretion balances intake with output so increased intake results in a large output and vice versa:

- **Osmolality** (the number of electrolytes and other molecules per kg/urine) measures the concentration or dilution. With dehydration, osmolality increases; with fluid retention, osmolality decreases. With kidney disease, urine is dilute and the osmolality is fixed.
- **Specific gravity** compares the weight of urine (weight of particles) to distilled water (1.000). Normal urine is 1.010-1.025 with normal intake. High intake lowers the specific gravity and low intake raises it. In kidney disease, it often does not vary.
- **Antidiuretic hormone** (ADH/vasopressin) regulates the excretion of water and urine concentration in the renal tubule by varying water reabsorption. When fluid intake decreases, blood osmolality rises and this stimulates release of ADH, which increases reabsorption of fluid to return osmolality to normal levels. ADH is suppressed with increased fluid intake, so less fluid is reabsorbed.

EVALUATING WOUNDS FOR ETIOLOGY

Wounds should be evaluated for etiology during the initial assessment to ensure proper treatment. Wounds can arise from a number of different causes:

- **Trauma**: Injuries resulting from accidents or other types of trauma may vary considerably with some resulting in extensive damage to bones, tissues, organs, and circulation. Additionally, the wounds may be contaminated. Each wound must be assessed individually for multiple factors.
- **Burns**: Burn wounds may be chemical or thermal and should be assessed according to the area, the percentage of the body burned, and the depth of the burn. First-degree burns are superficial and affect the epidermis. Second-degree burns extend through the dermis. Third degree burns affect underlying tissue, including vasculature, muscles, and nerves.
- **Infection**: An infected surgical or wound site can result in pain, edema, cellulitis, drainage, erosion of the sutures and ulceration of the tissue. Surgical sites must be assessed carefully and laboratory findings reviewed.

ELEMENTS OF WOUND ASSESSMENT

LOCATION AND SIZE

Wound location should be described in terms of anatomic position using landmarks (such as sternal notch, umbilicus, lateral malleolus), correct medical terminology, and directional terms:

- Anterior (in front)
- Posterior (behind)
- Superior (above)
- Inferior (below)

Wound size should be carefully described through actual measurement rather than association (the size of a dime). Measurements should be done with a disposable ruler in millimeters or centimeters. The current standard for measurement:

$$\text{Length} \times \text{width} \times \text{depth} = \text{dimension}$$

However, a clear description requires more detail. The measurement should be done at the greatest width and greatest length. More than 2 measurements may be needed if the wound is very irregularly shaped. The depth of the wound should be measured by inserting a sterile applicator and grasping or marking the applicator at skin level and then measuring the length below. Ideally, the wound should be photographed as well following protocols for photography.

WOUND BED TISSUE

Wound bed tissue should be described as completely as possible, including color and general appearance:

- **Granulation tissue** should be slightly granular in appearance and deep pink to bright red and moist, bleeding easily if disturbed.
- **Clean non-granular tissue** is smooth and deep pink or red and is not healing.
- **Hypergranulation** is excessive soft flaccid granulating tissue that is raised above the level of the periwound tissue, preventing proper epithelization, and may reflect excess moisture in the wound,.
- **Epithelization** should appear at wound edges first and then eventually cover the wound. It is dry and light pink or violet in color.

- **Slough** is necrotic tissue that is viscous, soft and yellow-gray in appearance and adheres to the wound.
- **Eschar** is hard dark brown or black leathery necrotic tissue that accumulates with death of the tissue.

WOUND MARGINS

Wound margins and the tissue surrounding the wound should be described carefully and with correct terminology:

- **Color** should be described using color descriptions and such terms as blanched, erythematous (red), or ecchymosed (purple, green, yellow).
- **Skin texture** may be normal, indurated (hardened), or edematous (swollen). Note if there is cellulitis or maceration evident.
- **Wound edges** may be diffuse (without clear margins), well defined, or rolled. A healing ridge may be evident if granulation has begun. Note if the wound is closed (as with a surgical incision) or open (as with dehiscence or ulcerations). Note if wound edges are attached or unattached (indicating undermining or tunneling).
- **Tunneling or undermining** should be assessed by probing the wound margins with a moist sterile cotton applicator, using clock face locators (toward the head is 12 o'clock, for example). Tunneling may be described as extending from 3 o'clock to 4 o'clock. A large area is usually described as undermining. The size should be measured or estimated as closely as possible.

DISTRIBUTION, DRAINAGE, AND ODOR

Distribution of lesions should be clearly delineated if there is more than one lesion over an area. The arrangement of the lesions can be helpful for diagnosis and treatments.

- Linear (in a line)
- Satellites (small lesions around a larger one)
- Diffuse (scattered freely over an area)

Drainage may vary considerably from nothing at all to copious outpourings of discharge.

- Serous drainage is usually clear to slightly yellow.
- Serosanguinous drainage is a combination of serous drainage and blood.
- Sanguinous drainage is bloody.
- Purulent discharge may be thick and milky, yellow, brownish, or green, depending upon the infective agent.

Odor requires more subjective assessment, but the odor and type of discharge together can provide useful information. Some infective agents, such as *Pseudomonas*, produce distinctive odors, which may be described in various ways: Musty, Foul, Sweet

PSYCHOSOCIAL ASSESSMENT

A **psychosocial assessment** should provide additional information to the physical assessment to guide the patient's plan of care and should include:

- Previous hospitalizations and experience with healthcare.
- Psychiatric history: Suicidal ideation, psychiatric disorders, family psychiatric history, history of violence and/or self-mutilation.
- Chief complaint: Patient's perception.

- Complementary therapies: Acupuncture, visualization, and meditation.
- Occupational and educational background: Employment, retirement, and special skills.
- Social patterns: Family and friends, living situation, typical activities, support system.
- Sexual patterns: Orientation, problems, and sex practices.
- Interests/abilities: Hobbies and sports.
- Current or past substance abuse: Type, frequency, drinking pattern, use of recreational drugs, and overuse of prescription drugs.
- Ability to cope: Stress reduction techniques.
- Physical, sexual, emotional, and financial abuse: Older adults are especially vulnerable to abuse and may be reluctant to disclose out of shame or fear.
- Spiritual/Cultural assessment: Religious/Spiritual importance, practices, restrictions (such as blood products or foods), and impact on health/health decisions.

MULTISYSTEM TRAUMA-TREATMENT PRIORITIZATION GUIDELINES

In order to give the trauma patient the best chance at survival, treatment must be appropriately **prioritized** and managed. Immediate priority should be given to maintaining the airway and ensuring adequate ventilation. Pre-hospital management should also include control of bleeding, prevention of shock, spine immobilization and neurological assessment. Upon arrival to the closest trauma center, the primary survey conducted by the healthcare trauma team is centered on determining which injuries are potentially life-threatening. Airway is the number one priority, followed by an assessment of hemodynamic status (assess for hypovolemia) and core body temperature (assess for hypothermia). Baseline data is also collected including laboratory studies, EKG, and radiologic testing. Treatment may include fluid resuscitation, the administration of blood products and surgical intervention (if indicated). Complications of multisystem trauma include disseminated intravascular coagulopathy, acute respiratory distress syndrome, renal failure, infection, compartment syndrome, dysrhythmias, and sepsis.

TYPES OF PAIN

NOCICEPTIVE PAIN

There are two **primary types of pain**: nociceptive (acute) pain and neuropathic pain although some people may have a combination. **Nociceptive** or acute pain is the normal nerve response to a painful stimulus. Trauma that results in nociceptive pain can cause severe inflammation and damage to nerve endings. Nociceptive pain usually correlates with extent and type of injury: the greater the injury, the greater the pain. It may be procedural pain (related to wound manipulation and dressing changes) or surgical pain (related to cutting of tissue). It may also be continuous or cyclic, depending upon the type of injury. This type of pain is usually localized to the area of injury and resolves over time as healing takes place. This type of pain is often described as aching or throbbing, but generally responds to analgesia. Uncontrolled, this type of pain can in time result in changes in the nervous system that lead to chronic neuropathic pain.

NEUROPATHIC PAIN

While nociceptive pain is acute, **neuropathic pain** is more chronic. **Neuropathic pain** occurs when there is a primary lesion in the nervous system or dysfunction related to damaged nerve fibers. Neuropathic pain may be associated with conditions such as diabetes, cancer, or traumatic injury to the nervous system. This type of pain is common in chronic wounds and is more often described as burning, stabbing, electric, or shooting pains. Often the underlying pathology causing the pain is not reversible. Pain may be visceral (diffuse or cramping pain of internal organs) caused by injuries to internal organs. It is also often diffuse rather than localized. It may also be somatic pain (involving muscles, skin, bones, and joints). Neuropathic pain is often more difficult to assess that nociceptive pain because the damage may alter normal pain responses. Neuropathic pain often responds better to antidepressants and anti-seizure medications than analgesics.

ADVERSE SYSTEMIC EFFECT OF PAIN

Acute pain causes **adverse systemic affects** that can negatively affect many body systems.

- **Cardiovascular**: Tachycardia and increased BP is a common response to pain, causing increased cardiac output and systemic vascular resistance. In those with pre-existing cardiovascular disease, such as compromised ventricular function, cardiac output may decrease. The increased myocardial need for oxygen may cause or worsen myocardial ischemia.
- **Respiratory**: Increased need for oxygen causes an increase in minute ventilation and splinting due to pain may compromise pulmonary function. If the chest wall movement is constrained, tidal volume falls, impairing the ability to cough and clear secretions. Bed rest further compromises ventilation.
- **Gastrointestinal**: Sphincter tone increases and motility decreases, sometimes resulting in ileus. There may be increased secretion of gastric acids, which irritate the gastric lining and can cause ulcerations. Nausea, vomiting, and constipation may occur. Reflux may result in aspiration pneumonia. Abdominal distension may occur.
- **Urinary**: Increased sphincter tone and decreased motility result in urinary retention.
- **Endocrine**: Hormone levels are affected by pain. Catabolic hormones, such as catecholamine, cortisol and glucagon increase and anabolic hormones, such as insulin and testosterone decrease. Lipolysis increases along with carbohydrate intolerance. Sodium retention can occur because of increased ADH, aldosterone, angiotensin, and cortisol. This in turn causes fluid retention and a shift to extracellular space.
- **Hematologic**: There may be reduced fibrinolysis, increased adhesiveness of platelets, and increased coagulation.
- **Immune**: Leukocytosis and lymphopenia may occur, increasing risk of infection.
- **Emotional**: Patients may become depressed, anxious, angry, depressed appetite, and sleep-deprived. This type of response is most common in those with chronic pain, who usually don't have typical systemic responses of those with acute pain.

PAIN ASSESSMENT IN CRITICAL CARE PATIENTS

Pain is subjective and may be influenced by the individual's pain threshold (the smallest stimulus that produces the sensation of pain) and pain tolerance (the maximum degree of pain that a person can tolerate). The most common current pain assessment tool for adults and pre-teens/adolescents is the 1-10 scale:

$$0 = \text{no pain.}$$
$$1 - 2 = \text{mild pain.}$$
$$3 - 5 = \text{moderate pain.}$$
$$6 - 7 = \text{severe pain.}$$
$$8 - 9 = \text{very severe pain.}$$
$$10 = \text{excruciating pain.}$$

However, there is more to pain assessment than a number on a scale. Assessment includes information about onset, duration, and intensity. Identifying what triggers pain and what relieves it can be very useful when developing a plan for pain management. Patients may show very different behavior when they are in pain: Some may cry and moan with minor pain, and others may exhibit little difference in behavior when truly suffering. Thus, judging pain by behavior can lead to the wrong conclusions.

PAINAD

Patients with cognitive impairment or inability to verbalize pain may not be able to indicate the degree of pain using the common 1-10 scale, even by using a face scale (FACES) with pictures of smiling to crying faces. **Pain Assessment in Advanced Dementia (PAINAD)** utilizes careful observation of nonverbal behavior to determine whether the patient is in pain:

- **Respirations:** Patients often have more Rapid and labored breathing as pain increases, with short periods of hyperventilation or Cheyne-Stokes respirations.
- **Vocalization:** Patients may remain negative in speech or speak quietly and reluctantly. They may moan or groan. As pain increases, they may call out, moan or groan loudly, or cry.
- **Facial expression:** Patients may appear sad or frightened, may frown or grimace, especially on activities that increase pain.
- **Body language:** Patients may be tense, fidgeting, pacing and as pain increases may become rigid, clench fists, or lie in fetal position. They may become increasingly combative.
- **Consolability:** Patients are less distractible or consolable with increased pain.

PAIN MANAGEMENT
PATIENT-CONTROLLED ANALGESIA

Patient-controlled analgesia (PCA) allows the patient to control administration of pain medication by pressing a button on an intravenous delivery system with a computerized pump. The device is filled with opioid (as prescribed) and must be programmed correctly and checked regularly to ensure that it is functioning properly and that controls are set. Current recommendations are that most patients that have an open (and some laparoscopic) surgical procedure use a PCA pump for pain control post operatively until they are tolerating fluids well orally. They may then be switched to oral pain medications. The most-commonly administered medications include morphine, meperidine, fentanyl, and hydromorphone. Most devices can be set to deliver continuous infusion of opioid as well as patient-controlled bolus. Each element must be set:

- **Bolus**: Determines the amount of medication received when the patient delivers a dose.
- **Lockout interval:** Time required between administrations of boluses.
- **Basal rate:** Rate at which continuous opioid is delivered per hour.
- **Limit** (usually set at 4 hours): Total amount of opioid that can be delivered in the preset time limit.

Important patient teaching includes instructing family members/others at bedside to never push the button for the patient (but can encourage when it is time). Also teach the patient that they cannot accidently overdose themselves to reduce fears and encourage use. Monitor for signs/symptoms of respiratory distress.

NON-ANALGESIC PAIN CONTROL MEASURES

Non-analgesic pain control measures begin with good communication between the patient and the healthcare provider and an assessment of the causes of pain, which can then be targeted for pain reduction.

- **Cleansing of wound**: Use normal saline and gentle flushing of wound rather than cytotoxic agents, such as antiseptics, which may cause burning and discomfort.
- **Peri-wound care**: Use skin sealants to protect intact skin from maceration and skin barriers over denuded skin.
- **Wound debridement**: Use autolysis when possible.

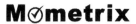

- **Dressings**: Select dressings with the goal of reducing pain as well as healing the wound. Moisture-retentive dressings often decrease pain. Avoid wet-to-dry dressings. Decrease frequency of dressing changes if possible.
- **Inflammation**: Elevate limb if indicated; provide medications to control.
- **Edema**: Elevate limbs and use compression dressings and sequential compression pumps as indicated.
- **Positioning**: Use body supports to stabilize wounds when possible. Use turning sheets. Try splinting or immobilizing a wound area.

GLASGOW COMA SCALE

The **Glasgow coma scale** (GCS) measures the depth and duration of coma or impaired level of consciousness and is used for post-operative assessment. The GCS measures three parameters: Best eye response, best verbal response, and best motor response, with scores ranging from 3 to 15:

- **Eye opening:**
  - 4: Spontaneous.
  - 3: To verbal stimuli.
  - 2: To pain (not of face).
  - 1: No response.
- **Verbal:**
  - 5: Oriented.
  - 4: Conversation confused, but can answer questions.
  - 3: Uses inappropriate words.
  - 2: Speech incomprehensible.
  - 1: No response.
- **Motor:**
  - 6: Moves on command.
  - 5: Moves purposefully respond pain.
  - 4: Withdraws in response to pain.
  - 3: Decorticate posturing (flexion) in response to pain.
  - 2: Decerebrate posturing (extension) in response to pain.
  - 1: No response.

Injuries/conditions are classified according to the total score: 3-8 Coma; ≤ 8 severe head injury; 9-12 moderate head injury; 13-15 mild head injury.

TRANSFUSIONS OF PRBC AND PLATELET CONCENTRATES

Blood components that are commonly used for transfusions include:

- **Packed red blood cells:** RBCs (250-300 mL per unit) should be warmed >30° (optimal 37°) before administration to prevent hypothermia and may be reconstituted in 50-100 mL of normal saline to facilitate administration. RBCs are necessary if blood loss is about 30% (1500-2000 mL) (Hgb ≤7). (Above 30% blood loss, whole blood may be more effective.) RBCs are most frequently used for transfusions.

- **Platelet concentrates:** Transfusions of platelets are used if the platelet count is <50,000 cells/mm³. One unit increases the platelet count by 5000-10,000 cells/mm³. Platelet concentrates pose a risk for sensitization reactions and infectious diseases. Platelet concentrate is stored at a higher temperature (20-24°) than RBCs. This contributes to bacterial growth, so it is more prone to bacterial contamination than other blood products and may cause sepsis. Temperature increase within 6 hours should be considered an indication of possible sepsis. ABO compatibility should be observed but is not required.

TRANSFUSIONS OF FFP AND CRYOPRECIPITATE

Blood components that are commonly used for transfusions include:

- **Fresh frozen plasma** (FFP) (obtained from a unit of whole blood frozen ≤6 hours after collection) includes all clotting factors and plasma proteins, so each unit administered increases clotting factors by 2-3%. FFP may be used for deficiencies of isolated factors, excess warfarin therapy, and liver-disease related coagulopathy. It may be used for patients who have received extensive blood transfusions but continue to hemorrhage. It is also helpful for those with antithrombin III deficiency. FFP should be warmed to 37°C prior to administration to avoid hypothermia. ABO compatibility should be observed if possible, but it is not required. Some patients may become sensitized to plasma proteins.
- **Cryoprecipitate** is the precipitate that forms when FFP is thawed. It contains fibrinogen, factor VIII, von Willebrand, and factor XIII. This component may be used to treat hemophilia A and hypofibrinogenemia.

TRANSFUSION-RELATED COMPLICATIONS

There are a number of **transfusion-related complications**, the reason that transfusions are given only when necessary. Complications include:

- **Infection**: Bacterial contamination of blood, especially platelets, can result in severe sepsis. A number of infective agents (viral, bacterial, and parasitic) can be transmitted although increased testing of blood has decreased rates of infection markedly. Infective agents include HIV, hepatitis C and B, human T-cell lymphotropic virus, CMV, WNV, malaria, Chagas' disease and variant Creutzfeldt-Jacob disease (from contact with mad cow disease).
- **Transfusion-related acute lung injury** (TRALI): This respiratory distress syndrome occurs ≤6 hours after transfusion. The cause is believed to be antileukocytic or anti-HLA antibodies in the transfusion. It is characterized by non-cardiogenic pulmonary edema (high protein level) with severe dyspnea and arterial hypoxemia. Transfusion must be stopped immediately and the blood bank notified. TRALI may result in fatality but usually resolves in 12-48 hours with supportive care.

Analysis

ARTERIAL BLOOD GASES

Arterial blood gases (ABGs) are monitored to assess effectiveness of oxygenation, ventilation, and acid-base status, and to determine oxygen flow rates. Partial pressure of a gas is that exerted by each gas in a mixture of gases, proportional to its concentration, based on total atmospheric pressure of 760 mm Hg at sea level. Normal values include:

- Acidity/alkalinity (pH): 7.35-7.45.
- Partial pressure of carbon dioxide ($PaCO_2$): 35-45 mm Hg.
- Partial pressure of oxygen (PaO_2): ≥80 mg Hg.

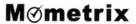

- Bicarbonate concentration (HCO_3^-): 22-26 mEq/L.
- Oxygen saturation (SaO_2): ≥95%.

The relationship between these elements, particularly the $PaCO_2$ and the PaO_2 indicates respiratory status. For example, $PaCO_2$ >55 and the PaO_2 <60 in a patient previously in good health indicates respiratory failure. There are many issues to consider. Ventilator management may require a higher $PaCO_2$ to prevent barotrauma and a lower PaO_2 to reduce oxygen toxicity.

> **Review Video: Blood Gases**
> Visit mometrix.com/academy and enter code: 611909

RED BLOOD CELL VALUES AND MORPHOLOGY

Red blood cells (RBCs or erythrocytes) are biconcave disks that contain hemoglobin (95% of mass), which carries oxygen throughout the body. The heme portion of the cell contains iron, which binds to the oxygen. RBCs live about 120 days after which they are destroyed and their hemoglobin is recycled or excreted. **Normal values** of red blood cell count vary by gender:

- Males >18 years: 4.5-5.5 million per mm^3.
- Females >18 years: 4.0-5.0 million per mm^3.

The most common disorders of RBCs are those that interfere with production, leading to various **types of anemia**:

- Blood loss
- Hemolysis
- Bone marrow failure

The **morphology of RBCs** may vary depending upon the type of anemia:

- Size: Normocytes, microcytes, macrocytes.
- Shape: Spherocytes (round), poikilocytes (irregular), drepanocytes (sickled).
- Color (reflecting concentration of hemoglobin: Normochromic, hypochromic.

LABORATORY TESTS

- **Hemoglobin:** Carries oxygen and is decreased in anemia and increased n polycythemia. Normal values:
  - Males >18 years: 14.0-17.46 g/dl.
  - Females >18 years: 12.0-16.0 g/dl.
- **Hematocrit:** Indicates the proportion of RBCs in a liter of blood (usually about 3 times the hemoglobin number). Normal values:
  - Males >18 years: 45-52%.
  - Females >18 years: 36-48%
- **Mean corpuscular volume (MCV):** Indicates the size of RBCs and can differentiate types of anemia. For adults, <80 is microcytic and >100 is macrocytic. Normal values:
  - Males > 18 years: 84-96 µm3.
  - Females >18 years: 76-96 µm3.
- **Reticulocyte count:** Measures marrow production and should rise with anemia. Normal values:
  - 0.5-1.5% of total RBCs.

- **C-reactive protein:** Increases with inflammation in the body.
  - Normal values: 2.6-7.6 µg/dL.
- **Erythrocyte sedimentation rate (sed rate):** a non-specific test that decreases with inflammation. Values vary according to gender and age:
  - <50: Males 0-15 mm/hr. Females 0-20 mm/hr.
  - >50: Males 0-20 mm/hr. Females 0-30 mm/hr.

WBC COUNT AND DIFFERENTIAL

White blood cell (leukocyte) count is used as an indicator of bacterial and viral infection. WBC is reported as the total number of all white blood cells. Normal WBC for adults: 4,800-10,000. Acute infection: 10,000+, 30,000 indicate a severe infection. Viral infection: 4,000 and below. **The differential** provides the percentage of each different type of leukocyte. An increase in the white blood cell count is usually related to an increase in one type and often an increase in immature neutrophils, known as bands, referred to as a "shift to the left", an indication of an infectious process:

- **Immature neutrophils (bands):**1-3%: Increase with infection.
- **Segmented neutrophils (segs):**50-62%: Increase with acute, localized, or systemic bacterial infections.
- **Eosinophils:** 0-3%: Decrease with stress and acute infection.
- **Basophils:** 0-1%: Decrease during acute stage of infection.
- **Lymphocytes:** 25-40%: Increase in some viral and bacterial infections.
- **Monocytes:** 3-7%: Increase during recovery stage of acute infection.

COAGULATION PROFILE

The following are elements of a coagulation profile:

- **Prothrombin time (PT):**
  - *Normal = 10 – 14 seconds.*
  - Increases with anticoagulation therapy, vitamin K deficiency, ↓prothrombin, DIC, liver disease, and malignant neoplasm.
- **Partial thromboplastin time (PTT)**
  - *Normal = 30 – 45 seconds.*
  - Increases with hemophilia A & B, von Willebrand's, vitamin deficiency, lupus, DIC, and liver disease.
- **Activated partial thromboplastin time (aPTT)**
  - *Normal = 21 – 35 seconds*
  - Similar to PTT, but decreases in extensive cancer, early DIC and after acute hemorrhage. Monitors heparin dosage.
- **Thrombin clotting time (TCT) or Thrombin time (TT)**
  - *Normal = 7 – 12 seconds (<21)*
  - Used most often to determine dosage of heparin. Prolonged with multiple myeloma, abnormal fibrinogen, uremia, and liver disease.
- **Bleeding time**
  - *Normal = 2 – 9.5 minutes (Ivy method on the forearm).*
  - Increases with DIC, leukemia, renal failure, aplastic anemia, von Willebrand's, some drugs, and alcohol.

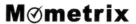

- **Platelet count**
  - ○ *Normal = 150,000 – 400,000 per microliter.*
  - ○ Increased bleeding <50,000 and increased clotting >750,000.

LIVER FUNCTION STUDIES
Liver Function Studies:

- Bilirubin – Shows the liver's ability to conjugate/excrete bilirubin:
  - ○ Direct 0.0-0.3 mg/dL.
  - ○ Total 0.0-0.9 mg/dL.
  - ○ Urine bilirubin 0.
- Total protein – Shows if the liver is producing normal protein levels:
  - ○ Total Protein7.0-7.5 g/dL.
  - ○ Albumin: 4.0-5.5 g/dL.
  - ○ Globulin: 1.7=3.3 g/dL.
  - ○ Albumin/globulin (A/G) ratio: 1.5:1 to 2.5:1.
- Alkaline phosphatase - Indicates biliary tract obstruction (in absence of bone disease)
  - ○ Alkaline phosphatase: 17-142 adults (varies with method).
- AST (SGOT)/ ALT (SGPT) - Increase in liver cell damage.
  - ○ AST: 10-40 units.
  - ○ ALT 5-35 units.
- Serum ammonia - Increases in liver failure.
  - ○ Ammonia: 150-250 mg/dL.

Will also see increase/abnormalities in lipids, cholesterol and clotting labs.

URINALYSIS
Urinalysis:

- **Color:** Pale yellow/ amber and darkens when urine is concentrated or other substances (such as blood or bile) or present.
- **Appearance:** Clear but may be slightly cloudy.
- **Odor:** Slight. Bacteria may give urine a foul smell, depending upon the organism.
- Some foods, such as asparagus, change odor.
- **Specific gravity:** 1.015 to 1.025. May increase if protein levels increase or if there is fever, vomiting, or dehydration.
- **pH:** Usually ranges from 4.5 - 8 with average of 5 - 6.
- **Sediment:** Red cell casts from acute infections, broad casts from kidney disorders, and white cell casts from pyelonephritis. Leukocytes > 10 per ml^3 are present with urinary tract infections.
- **Glucose, ketones, protein, blood, bilirubin, & nitrate:** Negative. Urine glucose may increase with infection (with normal blood glucose). Frank blood may be caused by some parasites and diseases but also by drugs, smoking, excessive exercise, and menstrual fluids. Increased red blood cells may result from lower urinary tract infections.
- **Urobilinogen:** 0.1-1.0 units.

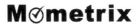

RENAL FUNCTION STUDIES

Renal Function:

- **Specific gravity:**1.015-1.025:Determines kidney's ability to concentrate urinary solutes.
- **Osmolality (urine):**350-900 mOsm/kg/24 hr :Shows early changes when kidney has difficulty concentrating urine.
- **Osmolality (serum):**275-295 mOsm/kg:Gives a picture of the amount of solutes in the blood.
- **Uric acid:**3.0-7.2 mg/dL:Increase with renal failure.
- **Creatinine clearance (24-hour):**75 to 125 mL/min.:Evaluates the amount of blood cleared of creatinine in 1 min. Approximates the GFR.
- **Serum creatinine:**0.6-1.2mg/dL:Increase with decreased renal fx, urinary tract obstruction, and nephritis.
- **Urine creatinine:**11-26 mg/kg/24 hr :Product of muscle breakdown. Increase with decreased renal fx.
- **Blood urea nitrogen (BUN):**7-8 mg/dL (8-20 mg/dL >age 60):Increase indicates impaired renal function, as urea is end product of protein metabolism.
- **BUN/creatinine ratio :**10:1:Increases with hypovolemia. With intrinsic kidney disease, the ratio is normal though increased BUN/Creatinine.

MEDICAL REASONING, DIAGNOSTIC REASONING, THERAPEUTIC REASONING, AND THERAPEUTIC UNCERTAINTY

Medical reasoning refers to the process by which clinicians gather data and information about a patient, and then use those data to arrive at a diagnosis and treatment plan. Diagnostic reasoning and therapeutic reasoning are subsets of medical reasoning; **diagnostic reasoning** is the information that is used to determine the most likely diagnosis, while **therapeutic reasoning** is the information used to determine what the best treatment is for that particular patient suffering from that particular disease. While the patient is undergoing treatment, it is necessary for the clinician to evaluate the patient's response to treatment on a regular basis. If it is not clear whether the patient is improving, or whether another treatment might be more beneficial, a degree of **therapeutic uncertainty** is introduced. There is also therapeutic uncertainty when the clinician is trying to decide which treatment option to use if the first treatment fails.

IMPORTANCE OF DATA GATHERING TO DIAGNOSTIC REASONING

The **gathering and recording of data** are of utmost importance to the diagnostic evaluation process. The history and physical section of the patient chart contains a wealth of information (ideally) and should always be taken into consideration when developing a care plan for the patient. Because any number of clinicians can add information to the patient chart (and because all of these clinicians will be reading this information), it is important to record all information clearly and in an organized manner. This can be a daunting task when considering all of the different sources of information, including the patient interview, family member interviews, previous charts, and lab results. By keeping this information clear and concise, errors are minimized, and the differential diagnosis is comprehensive.

SENSITIVITY AND SPECIFICITY IN RELATION TO DIAGNOSTIC TESTING

Some degree of error is inherent in almost all diagnostic testing. When ordering a diagnostic test for a patient, how confident can one be that the result will be accurate? The terms **sensitivity and specificity** are used to illustrate the accuracy of diagnostic tests. The sensitivity of a test refers to its ability to correctly identify patients who do have the disease. If a test is administered to 100 patients with diabetes, and all 100 patients test positive, the test is considered to have a sensitivity of 100%. If only 85 of those tested have a positive result, however, that means that the test has a false-negative rate of 15%, and a

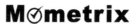

sensitivity of 85%. On the other hand, the specificity of a diagnostic test refers to its ability to identify patients who do not have the disease. If 100 nondiabetic patients are tested for diabetes, and 50 of them have a positive result, the test has a specificity of only 50%.

DIFFERENTIAL DIAGNOSIS PROCESS

The **differential diagnosis** is an important tool that allows the clinician to familiarize him or herself with the patient's condition, understand the condition, create an effective treatment plan, and follow the progress of the patient. To start, thoroughly examine the patient's chart, making a list of all of the abnormal test results and laboratory values. Add to this list all of the patient's complaints. Once this list is complete, organize the test results, labs, and complaints by anatomic location or organ system. After breaking the list down by organ site, look for any relationships between symptoms and/or results. Create another list of those data that seem to be related, and list all of the diseases or conditions that explain the findings, eliminating any that do not fit.

ANALYTICAL DECISION-MAKING

An **analytical decision** is one that is made after a systematic review and analysis of all factors involved in the decision; concentration and awareness are important in the analytical decision-making process. In contrast with an intuitive decision, the analytical decision takes longer to make, because it is not automatic. The analysis is based on an in-depth look at all factors, and is based on scientific evidence (in other words, it is based on the outcomes of previous similar situations). Because an analytical decision is based on scientific evidence and facts, the outcome of the decision has a high predictive value; this means that by looking at previous outcomes, it is possible to predict the current outcome. Because the clinician has so carefully reviewed all factors, he or she will most likely not experience the emotional anxiety associated with an intuitive decision.

INTUITIVE DECISION-MAKING

When a clinician makes an **intuitive decision**, he or she is making a decision not necessarily based on fact, but more so because it feels like the right decision. Of course, in most cases, one would not want a doctor making decisions this way, although in certain cases (say, a choice between 2 different types of treatment, each of which has the same general risks, or when all other options have been exhausted), it may be necessary. Although these decisions are not based on an analysis of the facts, there is something to be said about the so-called "gut instinct," which years of training and experience can hone. These decisions are made without spending a lot of time on the process of decision-making; though they are based on experience, the clinician may suffer some degree of anxiety about the decision and its outcome.

INFLUENTIAL FACTORS IN CLINICAL DECISION-MAKING PROCESS

Although one would like to think that there isn't much variation in the clinical decision-making process, this simply is not true. The process, of course, will differ depending on the patient, the differential diagnosis, and the clinician. The first variable to consider is the clinician. The way that the clinician conducts the clinical decision-making process is influenced by the knowledge base of the clinician, as well as the level of his experience, the ability he possesses to think both critically and creatively, and the confidence that he has in his ability to make educated decisions. The acuity level of the patient is also a factor in the clinical decision-making process, as is the length of the differential. A time stressor is placed on the clinician when the condition of the patient is critical, and when there are more diseases that must be eliminated from the differential. An element of stress may also exist if the clinician has a high number of patients, especially if he has multiple high-acuity patients.

QUESTIONS TO CONSIDER WHEN DEALING WITH DIAGNOSTIC AND THERAPEUTIC UNCERTAINTY

Diagnosis and subsequent treatment are not easily arrived at for every patient because every patient is different. The clinical presentation of a heart attack, for example, may include severe chest pain, sweating,

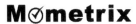

and nausea for one patient, and may have very mild, almost unnoticeable symptoms in another. **Diagnostic uncertainty** is especially prominent when dealing with diseases that have nonspecific symptoms; in these cases, it is important that the clinician recognize which of the possible diagnoses are life-threatening, and which are not. Ruling out the life-threatening possibilities should be higher on the clinician's list of priorities than the nonlife-threatening ones. Diagnostic testing, and subsequent treatment options, should also be evaluated according to the risks and benefits to the patient.

DEGREE OF CLINICAL UNCERTAINTY

Although the degree of uncertainty is somewhat dependent on the patient, the clinical setting can have an influence on the degree of uncertainty that the clinician is likely to encounter. For example, a clinic, such as a dermatology clinic, is a setting in which the degree of uncertainty is likely to be low; this is because the clinic is nonemergent, and because the clinic treats a specific, limited group of diseases with which the clinicians are very familiar. An urgent care clinic would fall somewhere in the middle, because although there is a wider range of diagnostic possibility, life-threatening emergencies are rarely encountered. An emergency room or a trauma center, on the other hand, sees a high degree of uncertainty; the clinicians see a wide range of diagnostic possibilities, and are expected to work at a fast pace.

APPROPRIATE EQUIPMENT TO PREPARE IN ANTICIPATION OF RECEIVING GUNSHOT VICTIM

The appropriate equipment needed for receiving a patient with a **gunshot wound** varies widely depending on the location of the wound, the severity, and complications (such as hemorrhage or pneumothorax). Intrabdominal injuries are common with gunshot wounds to the trunk, and penetrating chest trauma is associated with up to three-quarters of trauma-related mortality. The initial goal is to control bleeding and stabilize patient for surgical repair if needed. Equipment may include:

- Trauma tray (may differ from one facility to another).
- Thoracotomy tray and equipment for needle decompression.
- Chest tubes and underwater seal system.
- IV setup and IV fluids for resuscitation.
- Central line tray.
- Dressing supplies, tourniquet (for extremity wounds).
- Irrigating solutions (NS).
- Foley catheter setup.
- Ultrasound, imaging equipment.
- ET tube and ventilatory equipment.
- NG tube for gastric decompression.
- ECG and defibrillator.

APPROPRIATE EQUIPMENT TO PREPARE IN ANTICIPATION OF RECEIVING PATIENT WITH SEVERE OPEN FRACTURE

The appropriate equipment needed for receiving a patient with a **severe open fracture** depends on the location of the fracture and secondary injuries, such as to vasculature, muscles, and nerves. Patients with open fractures generally receive referral to an orthopedic specialist for surgical repair, so treatment in the trauma center may focus on controlling bleeding, preventing infection, and preparing the patient for surgery. Equipment needed may include:

- Blood administration setup.
- IV setup.

- Irrigating solutions (typically NS): initial cleaning may be carried out to remove obvious contaminants but extensive irrigation is often done in the operating room as part of cleaning and debriding the wound.
- Splint, appropriate to fracture site, is needed to stabilize the bones and prevent further injury.
- Tetanus prophylaxis if needed.
- Antibiotics (Cephalosporin for type 1 and type II fractures with addition of aminoglycoside is severely contaminated).
- Dressing supplies: Wound is usually covered with saline-soaked dressings until surgery.
- Imaging equipment (if portable in use).

Implementation

EFFECTS OF AGE ON SKIN

Age is an important consideration when evaluating the skin because the characteristics of the skin change as people age.

- An **infant**'s skin is thinner than an adult's because, while the epidermis is developed, the dermis layer is only about 60% of that of an adult and continues to develop after birth. The skin of premature infants is especially friable, allowing for transepidermal water loss and evaporative heat loss.
- During **adolescence**, the hair follicles activate and the thickness of the dermis decreases about 20% and epidermal turnover time increases, so healing slows.
- As people **continue to age**, Langerhans' cells decrease in number, making the skin more prone to cancer, and the inflammatory reactions decrease. The sweat glands, vascularity, and subcutaneous fat all decrease, interfering with thermoregulation and contributing to dryness and irritation of the skin. The epidermal-dermal junction flattens, resulting in skin prone to tearing. The elastin in the skin degrades with age and solar exposure. The thinning of the hypodermis can lead to pressure ulcers.

AGE-SPECIFIC NEEDS FOR INFANTS, CHILDREN, AND WOMEN OF CHILDBEARING AGE

Age-specific needs include:

- **Infants:** Most common injuries are to head and neck areas, and fractures most often of hand or arm. Bruises and head injuries should raise suspicion of abuse. Presence of bruises is often associated with other injuries. Infants should be naked for examination although diaper can be applied after examining genital and rectal areas.
- **Children**: Age-appropriate assessments must be conducted and protocols established for identifying children with possible abuse and reporting to appropriate authorities. When possible, parents should remain with children during assessment and treatments and assist with procedures, such as by holding the child during blood draws.
- **Females, childbearing age**: A suspicion of pregnancy should always be made with females of child-bearing age when considering medications and treatments that may result in damage to a fetus. The patient should be questioned about maternity status and use of birth control, when appropriate. In some cases, pregnancy testing may be indicated.

VASCULAR INTERVENTIONS

Vascular interventions are required when a patient has a condition that is decreasing blood flow to the limbs, causing ischemia-related damage. Conditions that require a vascular intervention include acute occlusion (embolus), severe unresponsive vascular disease, ruptured/dissecting aneurysm, damaged vessels, or congenital defect.

- **Bypass grafts:** The MD uses a harvested vein from another part of the body (saphenous usually) or synthetic graft to bypass the occlusion. Because veins have valves, they must be reversed or stripped of valves prior to attachment; however, synthetic grafts have a higher failure rate. A common peripheral bypass is the femoro-popliteal (Fem-pop) bypass, extending from the femoral artery around the blockage to the popliteal artery.
- **Embolectomy:** A catheter is inserted into the blocked artery and threaded through the thrombus. Then a balloon on the tip is inflated, and the physician removes the catheter, removing the clot with it.
- **Aortic Aneurysm Repair:** Intense procedure, requiring an open incision and the patient to be placed on cardiopulmonary bypass. The affected area is resected and replaced with a vascular or Dacron graft.

Nursing considerations: Monitor and control blood pressure carefully to protect patency and integrity of the grafts. Neurologic and renal function should also be carefully monitored, as emboli could block renal or cerebral artery. Frequent neuro, urine output, vascular and dressing checks.

Possible Complications: Pulmonary infection, graft-site infection, renal dysfunction, occlusion, hemorrhage, embolus/thrombus.

PERIPHERAL STENTS

Peripheral vascular stenting may be utilized as an intervention in the treatment of peripheral vascular insufficiency. Often performed in interventional radiology, the interventionalist uses balloon angioplasty to unblock the vessel under fluoroscopic guidance. A small balloon attached to a catheter is inserted into the occluded vessel and inflated to expand the arterial wall and compress the blockage. A small metal tube (stent) is then placed to support the vessel and maintain its patency. Stents are primarily made of stainless steel or a metal alloy. This intervention helps to restore circulation to the affected area and prevent restenosis of the vessel. There are different types of stents available based on the type of vessel affected and the type of lesion. Stenting may be used in both peripheral and coronary arteries.

- **Indications**: Stenting may be the initial choice of intervention in patients with iliac, renal, subclavian or carotid stenosis. Stenting may be indicated in patients with severe claudication, non-healing ulcers of the extremities, ischemic pain with rest and in patients who have a high operative risk. Peripheral stenting often results in shorter hospital stays and shorter recovery times in comparison with surgical intervention.
- **Complications**: Complications that may occur in patients undergoing peripheral stenting include: bleeding, infection, arterial spasm or rupture, dissection of the vessel, restenosis or thrombus formation within the vessel and intravascular fracture of the stent.

ARTERIAL LINE INSERTION

Indications for an **arterial line** include hemodynamic instability, frequent ABG monitoring, placement of IABP, monitoring arterial pressure, and medication administration when venous access cannot be obtained. Sterile technique is utilized for arterial line insertion. Insertions sites include radial (most common), femoral (second choice), brachial, or dorsalis pedis arteries. **Procedure**:

- Verify adequate perfusion and position:
  - Radial: Perform modified Allen test, and position wrist in dorsiflexion with armboard.

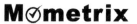

- o Femoral: Place patient in supine position with leg on insertion side slightly abducted and extended.
- Prep and drape. Apply 1% lidocaine if patient conscious.
- Over-wire catheter: Inserted into artery at 30-45° angle until blood returns, needle is removed, and catheter slightly advanced, wire inserted and advanced, catheter advanced over wire, wire removed, and catheter connected to transducer system.
- Over the needle catheter: Inserted at 30-45° degree angle and decreased to 10-15° angle when blood returns, catheter advanced into vessel, needle removed, and catheter connected to transducer.
- A small incision is made at insertion site and catheter sutured into place.

Complications include bleeding, coagulopathy, thrombosis (especially with larger catheters or smaller arteries), advanced atherosclerosis, and infection.

CENTRAL LINE INSERTION

Central lines allow rapid administration of large volumes of fluid, blood testing, and CVP measuring. Central lines may be placed into the internal jugular vein (right preferred), subclavian vein, or femoral vein (usually avoided). The insertion site is located through ultrasound. The patient is positioned, supine Trendelenburg (or legs elevated) for interior jugular, using sterile technique. Following skin prep, the CVC kit is placed on sterile field, opened, equipment prepared, and the insertion site again verified by probe (covered with sterile cover). Topical anesthetic (lidocaine) is administered and needle inserted with triangulation or spear method, always pulling back on plunger of syringe so that blood returns when entering the vein. The syringe is removed and guidewire inserted into needle ≤20 cm, needle removed, and wire position verified with ultrasound. A small incision is made at the insertion site and dilator applied over the wire and inserted about 2.5 to 3.5 cm. Catheter is placed over the wire and advanced into the vein (13 to 17 cm) and wire removed, lines flushed, and catheter sutured in place and dressing applied. Long (24 inch) PICCs may be inserted in the basilic or cephalic veins and advanced into central circulation.

PERICARDIOCENTESIS

Pericardiocentesis is done with ultrasound guidance to diagnose pericardial effusion or with ECG and ultrasound guidance to relieve cardiac tamponade. Pericardiocentesis may be done as treatment for cardiac arrest or with presentation of PEA with increased jugular venous pressure. Non-hemorrhagic tamponade may be relieved in 60-90% of cases, but hemorrhagic tamponade requires thoracotomy, as blood will continue to accumulate until the cause of the hemorrhage is corrected. Resuscitation equipment must be available, including a defibrillator, intravenous line in place, and cardiac monitoring:

- **Procedure:**
  - o Elevate chest 45° to bring heart closer to chest wall, pre-medicate with atropine and insert nasogastric tube if indicated.
  - o Cleanse skin with chlorohexidine or other appropriate cleanser
  - o After insertion of the needle using ultrasound guidance, the obturator is removed and a syringe attached for aspiration.
  - o The needle can often be replaced with a catheter after removal for drainage.
  - o Post procedure chest x-ray should be done to check for pneumothorax.
- **Possible Complications**: pneumo/hemothorax, coronary artery rupture, hepatic injury, dysrhythmias, false negative/positive aspiration.

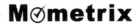

TRANSCUTANEOUS PACING

Transcutaneous pacing is used temporarily in an emergency situation to treat bradydysrhythmia that doesn't respond to medications (atropine) and results in hemodynamic instability. Generally, the patient provided oxygen and some sort of sedation before the pacing. The placement of pacing pads is usually one pacing pad (negative) is placed on the left chest, inferior to the clavicle, and the other (positive) on the left back, inferior to the scapula, so the heart is sandwiched between the two. Lead wires attach the pads to the monitor. The rate of pacing is usually set around 80 BPM. Current is increased slowly until capture occurs—a spiking followed by QRS sequence, then the current is readjusted downward if possible just to maintain capture, keeping it 5-10mA above the pacing threshold. Both demand and fixed modes are available, but demand mode is preferred.

CARDIOVERSION

Cardioversion is a timed electrical stimulation to the heart to convert a tachydysrhythmia (such as atrial fibrillation) to a normal sinus rhythm. Usually anticoagulation therapy is done for at least 3 weeks prior to elective cardioversion to reduce the risk of emboli and digoxin is discontinued for at least 48 hours prior. During the procedure, the patient is usually sedated and/or anesthetized. Electrodes in the form of gel-covered paddles or pads are placed in the anteroposterior position, and then connected by leads to a computerized ECG and cardiac monitor with a defibrillator. The defibrillator is synchronized with the ECG so that the electrical current is delivered during ventricular depolarization (QRS). The timing must be precise in order to prevent ventricular tachycardia or ventricular fibrillation. Sometimes, drug therapy is used in conjunction with cardioversion; for example, antiarrhythmics (Cardizem®, Cordarone®) may be given before the procedure to slow the heart rate.

- **Arrhythmia:** Beginning Monophasic Shock/Beginning Biphasic Shock
  - *A fib:* 50-100 J/ 25 J
  - *A flutter:*25-50 J/ 15 J
  - *Vtach* (monomorphic asymptomatic):100-200 J / 50 J

EMERGENCY DEFIBRILLATION

Emergency defibrillation is non-synchronized shock which is given to treat acute ventricular fibrillation, pulseless ventricular tachycardia, or polymorphic ventricular tachycardia with a rapid rate and decompensating hemodynamics. Defibrillation can be given at any point in the cardiac cycle. It causes depolarization of myocardial cells, which can then repolarize to regain a normal sinus rhythm. Defibrillation delivers an electrical discharge through pads/paddles. In an acute care setting, the preferred position to place the pads is the anteroposterior position. In this position one pad is placed to the right of the sternum, about the second to third intercostal space and the other pad is placed between the left scapula and the spinal column. This decreases the chances of damaging implanted devices, such as pacemakers, and this positioning has also been shown to be more effective for external cardioversion (if indicated at some point during resuscitation). There are two main types of defibrillator shock waveforms, monophasic and biphasic. Biphasic defibrillators deliver a shock one direction for half of the shock, and then in the return direction for the other half, making them more effective, and able to be used at lower energy levels. Monophasic defibrillation is given at 200-360 J and biphasic defibrillation is given at 100-200 J.

AIRWAY DEVICES

Airways are used to establish a patent airway and facilitate respirations:

- **Oropharyngeal**: This plastic airway curves over the tongue and creates space between the mouth and the posterior pharynx. It is used for anesthetized or unconscious patients to keep tongue and epiglottis from blocking the airway.

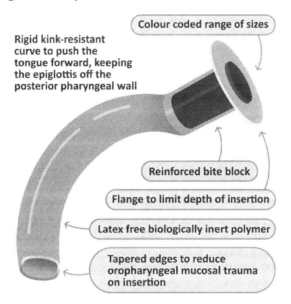

Colour coded range of sizes

Rigid kink-resistant curve to push the tongue forward, keeping the epiglottis off the posterior pharyngeal wall

Reinforced bite block

Flange to limit depth of insertion

Latex free biologically inert polymer

Tapered edges to reduce oropharyngeal mucosal trauma on insertion

- **Nasopharyngeal** (trumpet): This smaller flexible airway is more commonly used in conscious patients and is inserted through one nostril, extending to the nasopharynx. It is commonly utilized in patients who need frequent suctioning.

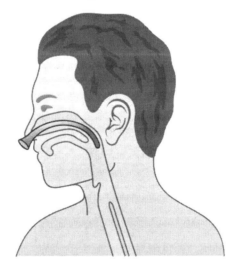

- **Tracheostomy tubes**: Tracheostomy may be utilized for mechanical ventilation. Tubes are inserted into the opening in the trachea to provide a conduit and maintain the opening. The tube is secured with ties around the neck. Because the air entering the lungs through the tracheostomy bypasses the warming and moistening effects of the upper airway, air is humidified through a room humidifier or through delivery of humidified air through a special mask or mechanical ventilation. If the tracheostomy is going to be long-term, eventually a stoma will form at the site and the tube can be removed.

ESOPHAGEAL-TRACHEAL COMBITUBE®

The **esophageal tracheal Combitube®** (ETC) is an intermediate airway that contains two lumens and can be inserted into either the trachea or the esophagus (≤91%). The twin-lumen tube has a proximal cuff providing a seal of the oropharynx and a distal cuff providing a seal about the distal tube. Prior to insertion, the Combitube® cuffs should be checked for leaks (15 ml of air into distal and 85 ml of air into proximal). The patient should be non-responsive and with absent gag reflex with head in neutral position. The tube is passed along the tongue and into the pharynx, utilizing markings on the tube (black guidelines) to determine depth by aligning the ETC with the upper incisors or alveolar ridge. Once in place the distal cuff is inflated (10-15 ml) and then placement in the trachea or esophagus should be determined, so the proper lumen for ventilation can be used. The proximal cuff is inflated (usually to 50-75 ml) and ventilation begun. Capnogram should be used to confirm ventilation.

TRACHEAL INTUBATION

Endotracheal intubation is often necessary with respiratory failure for control of hypoxemia, hypercapnia, hypoventilation, and/or obstructed airway. Equipment should be assembled and tubes and connections checked for air leaks with a 10 ml syringe. The mouth and/or nose should be cleaned of secretions and suctioned if necessary. The patient should be supine with the patient's head level with the lower sternum of the clinician. With orotracheal/endotracheal intubation, the clinician holds the laryngoscope (in left hand) and inserts it into right corner of mouth, the epiglottis is lifted and the larynx exposed. A thin flexible intubation stylet may be used and the endotracheal tube (ETT) (in right hand) is inserted through the vocal cords and into the trachea, cuff inflated to minimal air leak (10 ml initially until patient stabilizes), and placement confirmed through capnometry or esophageal detection devices. The correct depth of insertion is verified: 21 cm (female), 23 cm (male). After insertion, the tube is secured.

CONFIRMING CORRECT PLACEMENT OF ENDOTRACHEAL TUBES

There are a number of methods to confirm correct placement of **endotracheal tubes**. Clinical assessment alone is not adequate.

- **Capnometry** utilizes an end-tidal CO_2 (ETCO$_2$) detector that measures the concentration of CO_2 in expired air, usually through pH sensitive paper that changes color (commonly purple to yellow). The capnometer is attached to the ETT and a bag-valve-mask (BVM) ventilator attached. The patient is provided 6 ventilations and the CO_2 concentration checked.
- **Capnography** is attached to the ETT and provides a waveform graph, showing the varying concentrations of CO_2 in real time throughout each ventilation (with increased CO_2 on expiration) and can indicate changes in respiratory status.
- **Esophageal detection devices** fit over the end of the ETT so that a large syringe can be used to attempt to aspirate. If the ETT is in the esophagus, the walls collapse on aspiration and resistance occurs whereas the syringe fills with air if the ETT is in the trachea. A self-inflating bulb (Ellick® device) may also be used.
- **Chest X-ray** provides visual confirmation of placement.

INSERTION AND MANAGEMENT OF CHEST TUBES

Chest tubes with a closed drainage system are usually left in place after thoracic surgery or pneumothorax to drain air or fluid. Nursing interventions during insertion include ensuring the patient receives adequate pain control, attending to sterile technique, assisting physician with suturing as needed, attaching the tube to the chest tube drainage device, placing an occlusive dressing, and confirming placement.

Chest tube drainage systems have 3 major parts: suction control, water seal, and a chamber for collection. The system should have no bubbling in the water seal area, but a subtle rise and fall of the water seal corresponding with respirations, and gentle bubbling in the suction control chamber.

Nursing interventions after chest tube is in place: In most circumstances, report drainage >100 mL/hr, assess tubing after position changes for occlusion, maintain sterile dressing, avoid stripping the tubing, and assessing the insertion site for drainage or crepitus, the tubing, the patency of the entire system, and the output (including color, amount, and any other traits). The nurse should be knowledgeable about specimen collection, replacing the system, and dealing with clots.

TENSION PNEUMOTHORAX AND NEEDLE DECOMPRESSION

A **tension pneumothorax** may result from chest trauma that results in laceration of a lung, allowing air to leak into the pleural space but not to escape. Indications include dyspnea, anxiety, chest pain, subcutaneous emphysema, jugular venous distention (not evident with hypovolemia), hyperresonance and decreased or absent breath sounds on affected side. A tracheal shift and hyperexpansion on the unaffected side may be evident. Needle decompression may be used as treatment for tension pneumothorax if the patient's hemodynamic status remains stable. Procedure:

- Provide supplemental oxygen and position patient in supine position.
- Utilize large bore (10-14 gauge) angiocatheter at least 8 cm in length.
- Cleanse the insertion site with antiseptic, such as alcohol swabs.
- Insert the needle perpendicular to the skin at the midclavicular line in the second or third intercostal space or at the anterior axillary line at the third or fourth intercostal space (making sure to position the needle over the ribs instead of under where neurovascular bundles are located).
- Advance the catheter until air is felt at distal end or the full length has been inserted, remove needle, leave catheter in place and secure with adhesive.

THORACENTESIS

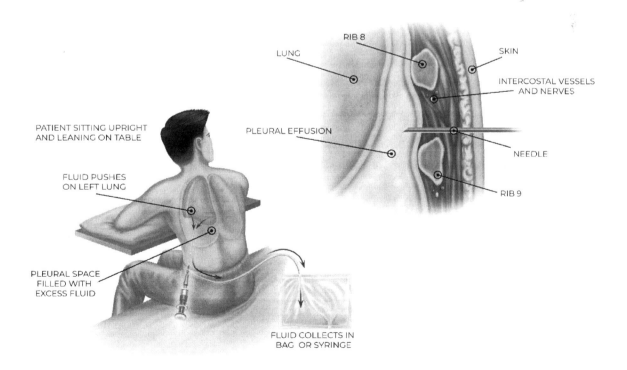

PATIENT SITTING UPRIGHT AND LEANING ON TABLE

FLUID PUSHES ON LEFT LUNG

PLEURAL SPACE FILLED WITH EXCESS FLUID

PLEURAL EFFUSION

LUNG

RIB 8

SKIN

INTERCOSTAL VESSELS AND NERVES

NEEDLE

RIB 9

FLUID COLLECTS IN BAG OR SYRINGE

A **thoracentesis** (aspiration of fluid or air from pleural space) is done to make a diagnosis, relieve pressure on the lung caused by pleural effusion, or instill medications. A chest x-ray is done prior to the procedure. A sedative may be given. The patient is in sitting position, leaning onto a padded bedside stand, straddling a chair with head supported on the back of the chair, or lying on the opposite side with the head of the bed elevated 30-45° to ensure that fluid remains at the base. The patient should avoid coughing or moving during the procedure. The chest x-ray or ultrasound determines needle placement. After a local anesthetic is administered, a needle (with an attached 20-ml syringe and 3-way stopcock with tubing and a receptacle) is advanced intercostally into the pleural space. Fluid is drained, collected, examined, and measured. The needle is removed and a pressure dressing applied. A chest x-ray is done to ensure there is no pneumothorax. The patient is monitored for cough, dyspnea, and hypoxemia.

BEDSIDE OPEN THORACOTOMY

A **bedside open thoracotomy** may be indicated for thoracic injuries although survival rates after penetrating trauma (gunshot and stab wounds) are better than after blunt trauma. Indications include pulselessness after witnessed cardiac activity, hypotension (systolic BP <70 mm Hg) despite resuscitation attempts, and >1500 mL blood returned from chest tube. Best outcomes are achieved if the open thoracotomy is done within 10-15 minutes after trauma. Contraindications include lack of witnessed cardiac activity, nontraumatic cardiac arrest, severe traumatic brain injury, and severe multisystem injuries. Procedure:

- Intubate patient and provide procedure sedation.
- Utilize sterile procedure (sterile PPE, drapes) and thoracotomy tray.
- Position patient supine with elevation (towels) under left scapula and left arm placed above the head.
- Prep chest and drape to prepare for anterolateral incision (usually left side).
- Carry out pericardiocentesis if cardiac tamponade present.
- *Note*: Descending aorta may be clamped to control hemorrhage or redistribute blood.
- *Note*: Cardiac wound may be sutured and/or internal cardiac massage carried out.

DRAINS

The following are the different types of drains a patient may have, including pertinent nursing considerations:

- **Simple drains** are latex or vinyl tubes of varying sizes/length. They are usually placed through a stab wound near the area of involvement.
- **Penrose drains** are flat, soft rubber/latex tubes placed in surgical wounds to drain fluid by gravity and capillary action.
- **Sump drains** are double-lumen or tri-lumen tubes (with a third lumen for infusions). The multiple lumen produce venting when air enters the inflow lumen and forces drainage out of the large lumen.
- **Percutaneous drainage catheter** is inserted into wound to provide continuous drainage for infection/fluid collection. Irrigation of the catheter may be required to maintain patency. Skin barriers and pouching systems may also be necessary.
- **Closed drainage systems** use low-pressure suction to provide continuous gravity drainage of wounds. Drains are attached to collapsible suction reservoirs that provide negative pressure. The nurse must remember to always re-establish negative pressure after emptying these drains. There are two types in frequent use:
  - ***Jackson-Pratt®*** *is* a bulb-type drain that is about the size of a lemon. A thin plastic drain from the wound extends to a squeeze bulb that can hold about 100ml of drainage.

- ○ ***Hemovac®*** is a round drain with coiled springs inside that are compressed after emptying to create suction. The device can hold up to 500 ml of drainage.

TROUBLE-SHOOTING PROBLEMS RELATED TO ENTERAL FEEDINGS

Feeding tubes are commonly found in the critical care setting, as many patients are intubated and unable to take oral nutrition or medication. General maintenance involves checking placement before flushing anything into tube (prevents aspiration), flushing the tubes with ≥30cc water before and after use, and every 4 hours. Never crush enteric-coated medications, and keep the HOB ≥ 30° at all times during feeding. **Complications** include:

- **Vomiting / aspiration:** Caused by incorrect placement, gastric emptying, formula intolerance.
  - ○ Tx: Confirm placement by checking pH (preferred to air bolus); Delay feeding one hour and check residual volume before resuming. Refrigerate formula, check expiration, use only for 24 hours.
- **Diarrhea:** Caused by rapid feeding, antibiotics/medications, intolerance of formula or hypertonic formula, tube migration.
  - ○ Tx: ↓ rate of feeding, evaluate medications, avoid hanging feedings ≥ 8 hours, add fiber or decrease sodium in feed.
- **Displacement of Tube:**
  - ○ Tx: NG tube- replace using other nostril, only if not surgically placed. G-tube/J-tube: cover site and notify physician. Prevention: secure all tubes with appropriate device, mark placement to identify migration.
- **Tube Occlusion:**
  - ○ Tx: Check for kinks/obvious problems. Aspirate fluid and instill warm water and aspirate to loosen occlusion. Physician may order enzyme or sodium bicarb solution.

TPN

Total parenteral nutrition (TPN) is an intravenous hypertonic solution containing glucose, fat emulsion, protein, minerals, and vitamins. TPN is generally given through a central line (PICC if short-term), and used only when other methods of nutrition are not feasible.

Nursing Considerations:

- **Infection prevention**: Use aseptic technique for feedings and dressing changes; change solution, filter, and tubing every 24 hours, discard cloudy solutions and monitor site for signs of infection.
- **Risk of embolus/contamination**: Use micropore filter (TPN without fat emulsion) or 1.2-micron filter (TPN with fat emulsion); can add heparin to solution. Never infuse any medication or product in same line as TPN; cannot draw blood from this line either.
- **Malnutrition and Electrolytes**: Check daily weight; BMP and CBC 3x a week until stable, then weekly. Check label and ingredients before administration; watch for signs of fluid overload. Cloudy blood specimen could indicate hyperlipidemia; also risk of hyper-ammonemia (asterix, AMS) and azotemia (dehydration, ↑BUN).
- **Hyper/Hypoglycemia**: Initiate slowly, increasing rate over 24-48hrs. NEVER "catch-up" rate if there is a delay/pause in feeding; only administer with a pump and do not change rate without order. If bag runs out, hang a bag of D10W until new bag can be obtained. Monitor BG every 4-6 hours; may use sliding scale insulin.

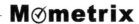

CRRT

Continuous renal replacement therapy (CCRT) circulates the blood by hydrostatic pressure through a semipermeable membrane. It is used in critical care and can be instituted quickly:

- **Continuous arteriovenous hemofiltration** (CAVH) circulates blood from an artery (usually the femoral) to a hemofilter using only arterial pressure and not a blood pump. The filtered blood is then returned to the patient's venous system, often with added fluids to offset those lost. Only the fluid in filtered.
- **Continuous arteriovenous hemodialysis** (CAVHD) is similar to CAVH except that dialysate circulates on one side of the semipermeable membrane to increase clearance of urea.
- **Continuous venovenous hemofiltration** (CVVH) pumps blood through a double-lumen venous catheter to a hemofilter, which returns the blood to the patient in the same catheter. It provides continuous slow removal of fluid, is better tolerated with unstable patients, and does not require arterial access.
- **Continuous venovenous hemodialysis** is similar to CVVH but uses a dialysate to increase clearance of uremic toxins.

COMPLICATIONS ASSOCIATED WITH HEMODIALYSIS AND PERITONEAL DIALYSIS

There are many **complications** associated with dialysis, especially when used for long-term treatment:

- **Hemodialysis***:* Long-term use promotes atherosclerosis and cardiovascular disease. Anemia and fatigue are common as are infections related to access devices or contamination of equipment. Some experience hypotension and muscle cramping during treatment. Dysrhythmias may occur. Some may exhibit dialysis disequilibrium from cerebral fluid shifts, causing headaches, nausea and vomiting, and alterations of consciousness.
- **Peritoneal dialysis:** Most complications are minor, but it can lead to peritonitis, which requires removal of the catheter if antibiotic therapy is not successful in clearing the infection within 4 days. There may be leakage of the dialysate around the catheter. Bleeding may occur, especially in females who are menstruating as blood is pulled from the uterus through the fallopian tubes. Abdominal hernias may occur with long use. Some may have anorexia from feeling of fullness or sweet taste in mouth from absorption of glucose.

CLIPPING FOR TREATMENT OF ANEURYSM

Surgical clipping of a ruptured or large, unstable **aneurysm** is necessary because of the danger of rebleeding, 4% in the first 24 hours and 1-2% each day for the next month. Mortality rates with rebleeding are about 70%. Surgical repair is usually done within 48 hours. Clipping may be done prophylactically to prevent rupture. Clipping is done to secure the aneurysm without impairing circulation. Typically, a craniotomy is done and an incision is made into the brain to access the site of the aneurysm. When bleeding is controlled, a small spring-like clip (or sometimes multiple clips) is placed about the neck of the aneurysm. The bulging part of the aneurysm is drained with a needle to make sure that it does not refill and angiography may be done to ensure patency of the artery that feeds the aneurysm. It is possible during surgery for a clot to break away from the aneurysm with resultant extensive hemorrhage. Neurological damage may occur related to surgical manipulation, especially if access is difficult. Post-op monitoring includes frequent neurological checks – sometimes every hour, checking for s/s of stroke, hemorrhage or cerebral edema/ increased ICP. An angiogram may be performed after surgery to confirm placement of clips and ensure there are no leaks.

EMBOLIZATION FOR TREATMENT OF ANEURYSM OR AVM

Embolization is a minimally-invasive method that is an alternative to clipping for some aneurysms and is also used for AVMs. There are different types of embolization, but all use percutaneous transfemoral catheterization and fluoroscopy. The catheter is fed through the femoral and carotid artery to the area requiring repair:

- AVM repair introducing small silastic beads or glue into the feeder vessels, allowing blood flow to carry the material to the site. This may also be done prior to surgical repair.
- AVM or aneurysm repair placing one or more detachable balloons into the aneurysm or an AVM and inflating it with a liquid polymerizing agent that solidifies.
- Aneurysm repair with endovascular coiling involves feeding very small platinum coils through the catheter to fill the aneurysm.

Results of endovascular coiling have been very positive, with risk of death or disability at one year over 22% lower than those treated with clipping although distal ischemia related to emboli is a possible complication.

CRANIOTOMIES

Craniotomies for tumors or other surgical repair (AVMs, aneurysms) are increasingly done with micro-endoscopic equipment, but the surgical opening must be large enough to allow access and the use of necessary instruments. Procedures vary widely according to the reason for craniotomy, the type of tumor, and the age and condition of the patient. Direct craniotomies through the skull are needed in some instances, but newer approaches, including transnasal and transsphenoidal endoscopy are used when possible. Some areas of the brain are not accessible with craniotomy, but may be accessible through stereotactic radiosurgery with Gamma Knife® or CyberKnife®. Stereotactic radiosurgery is often used as a secondary treatment after primary removal of tumor for regrowth or residual tumor. Radiosurgery may be fractionated and given in a series of treatments. These non-invasive treatments are usually done while adults are awake.

POSTOPERATIVE CARE FOR CRANIOTOMY PATIENT

In the post-operative period immediately following a **craniotomy**, the patient must be observed carefully for any complications or changes in condition:

- Intracranial pressure monitoring.
- Positioning: Head is usually positioned in midline, neutral position. The head of bed is elevated 30-45° for supratentorial surgery and is flat or only slightly elevated for infratentorial surgery.
- Fluid balance (intake and output).
- Wound care includes observation for swelling, drainage, and emptying and measuring any drainage devices (usually bulb drains) left in place.
- Oximetry and ABGs to ensure proper oxygenation.
- Analgesia and antiemetics are given routinely to maintain comfort and prevent stress/increased ICP from vomiting.
- Corticosteroids to reduce postoperative swelling.
- Anticoagulants (heparin) to prevent clotting.
- Monitor laboratory status:
  - Complete blood count to observe for blood loss/ infection.
  - Electrolyte levels, especially observing for hyponatremia and/or hyperkalemia.
  - Blood glucose level (may elevate with corticosteroids).
- Monitor thermoregulation and prevent hyperthermia.
- Anti-thromboembolism measures: Compression stockings or intermittent pneumatic compression.

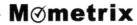

MONITORING DEVICES FOR ABDOMINAL COMPARTMENT SYNDROME

Measurement of **intra-abdominal pressure** is by attaching a pressure transducer or water-column manometer to a Foley catheter in the bladder because bladder pressure correlates with abdominal pressure. The patient should be in supine flat position if possible. The bladder must be empty for accurate measurement. The catheter should be clamped and transducer zeroed at the iliac crest along the midaxillary line. Then, 2 to 25 mL (usually about 10 mL for critically ill) of fluid is injected into the bladder and left in place for 30 to 60 seconds before the reading pressure following a patient expiration. Compartment pressures should be <30 mm Hg and the difference between diastolic BP and compartment pressure should be >30 mm Hg. Intraabdominal pressure may also be checked with an indwelling NG tube. If risk for compartment syndrome exists, the wound should not be closed. Sudden release of pressure and reperfusion may cause acidosis, vasodilation, and cardiac arrest, so the patient should be given crystalloid solutions before decompression.

MONITORING DEVICES FOR EXTREMITY COMPARTMENT SYNDROME

Signs of **extremity compartment syndrome** include the 5 P's: (1) pain that is severe and out of proportion to injury, (2) paresthesia, (3) pallor, (4) paresis, and (5) pulse deficit. Pressure is typically measured with a device specially intended for measurement although it can also be measured by attaching a manometer to a needle and syringe. The procedure with the Stryker intercompartmental pressure monitor device includes:

- First, the skin is cleansed with antiseptic and a local anesthetic administered.
- The pressure monitor device (or similar) contains a 3 mL syringe, a chamber and needle that connect to the syringe, and a pressure monitor into which the syringe is placed.
- Air is purged from the chamber and needle with the saline.
- The syringe is placed into the pressure monitoring device.
- The device is turned on, zeroed automatically by pressing the "zero" button.
- The needle is inserted into the compartment.
- Once the needle is inserted, about 0.3 mL of NS is injected and the device automatically records the compartment pressure. If over 30 mm Hg, a fasciotomy is usually needed.

PELVIC STABILIZER

Pelvic stabilizers are used to prevent excessive bleeding associated with pelvic fractures, to maintain the bones in correct position, and to prevent further damage. Maintaining pressure and reducing the fracture often reduces bleeding. Various methods of stabilizing the pelvis may be employed, including the sheet wrap method in which a sheet is folded, center under the patient, wrapped tightly about the pelvis, and secured. The pneumatic anti-shock garment (PASG) is indicated for hypovolemic shock, and hypotension associated with and for stabilization of pelvic and bilateral femur fractures. PASG is contraindicated with respiratory distress, pulmonary edema), pregnancy (2-3rd trimesters), heart failure, myocardial infarction, stroke, evisceration, abdominal or leg impalement, head injuries, and uncontrolled bleeding above the garment. Another device is the SAM pelvic sling, which has a wide band that fits under and about the pelvis and lateral hips and a belt anteriorly that allows adjustment.

IMMOBILIZATION DEVICES

Immobilization devices include:

- **Cervical collar**: Support the head to prevent spinal cord injury with suspected injury to cervical vertebrae.
- **Cervical extrication splints**: Short board used to immobilize and protect the head and neck during extrication.

- **Backboards**: Used to immobilize the spine to prevent further injury to spinal cord. Both long and short spine boards are available in a number of different shapes and sizes.
- **Full-body splints** (such as vacuum mattress splint): Provide cushioned support to maintain body alignment.
- **Various types of splints for extremities**: Include rigid (should be padded), non-rigid (moldable), traction, and air (pneumatic devices) as well as the use of blankets, rolled towels, sheets, and pillows to maintain position. Traction splints are used for fractured femurs to keep bones in position.
- **Pneumatic anti-shock garment** (PASG, shown below): Provides pressure on lower extremities and abdomen and is used to control hemorrhage and shock to prevent pooling of blood in extremities and return blood to general circulation. Often used for pelvic fractures, but may increase risk of internal hemorrhage.

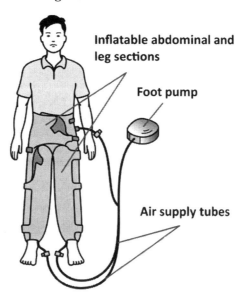

Inflatable abdominal and leg sections

Foot pump

Air supply tubes

TOURNIQUETS

Tourniquets are used to control hemorrhage in an extremity and should be applied immediately with arterial bleeds or if pressure does not stop bleeding. Commonly used tourniquets include adjustable bands that are tightened and secured, and then include a windlass handle twisted until blood flow stops and the handle secured. Another type is a wide elastic band that is stretched, wrapped about the extremity tightly a number of times and secured. Blood pressure cuffs may also be used to apply pressure if standard tourniquets are not available. Regardless of the type, the tourniquet should be placed as high on the extremity as possible (avoiding joints) and the date and time of placement documented (on the tourniquet if possible). Tourniquets may be contraindicated with DVT, Reynaud's disease, crushing injuries, sickle cell disease, severe peripheral arterial disease, and open lower extremity fractures. Risks include damage to muscles, nerves, and vessels as well as increased risk of amputation. However, the first priority is always to prevent exsanguination.

INTRAOSSEOUS INFUSION

Intraosseous (IO) infusion is an alternative to IV access for neonates, pediatric emergencies, and adult emergencies when rapid temporary access is necessary or when peripheral or vascular access can't be achieved. It is often used in pediatric cardiac arrest. Because yellow marrow replaces red marrow, access in those older than 5 is more difficult. Preferred sites are based on age, though across all ages, the **proximal tibia is preferred**. Additional sites include:

- 0-1: Distal femur
- 1-12: Distal tibia or fibula
- 12-18: Distal tibia or fibula, sternum
- 18 and older: Distal tibia or fibula, proximal humerus, sternum

IO infusion is used to administer fluids and anesthesia and to obtain blood samples. Equipment requires a special needle (13-20 gauge) as standard needles may bend. The bone injection gun (BIG) with a loaded spring facilitates insertion. The FAST needle is intended for use in the sternum of adults and prevents accidental puncture of the thoracic cavity. Knowledge of bony landmarks and correct insertion angle and site is important. The position is confirmed by aspiration of 5-10 mL of blood and marrow before infusion.

AUTOTRANSFUSION

Autotransfusion (autologous blood transfusion) is collecting of the patient's blood and reinfusing it. This is lifesaving with severe bleeding if other donor blood is not available. Blood in trauma cases is usually collected from a body cavity, such as pleural (hemothorax with ≥1500 mL blood) or peritoneal space (rare). Autotransfusion is contraindicated if malignant lesions are present in area of blood loss, contamination of pooled blood, or wounds >4-6 hours old. Commercial collection/transfusion kits (Pleur-Evac®, Thora-Klex®) are available but blood can be collected through the chest tube into a sterile bottle, which is then disconnected and connected to IV tubing for infusion, OR the blood in the bottle may be transferred to a blood collection bag for use. Commercial kits use either a chest tube or suction tube to withdraw blood and provide specific procedures. Blood is filtered. Heparin is not routinely used but citrate phosphate dextrose (CPD) (25-70 mL/500 mL blood) is often added to the aspirant to prevent clotting. Complications from autotransfusion are rare.

FLUID RESUSCITATION FOR BURN INJURIES

Burn victims are at risk for hypovolemia and electrolyte imbalances because of loss of body fluids through burned areas. **Fluid resuscitation** is indicated with burns of 20% or more of total body surface area (TBSA) burned. Lactated Ringers IV solution is used instead of NS, which can lead to hypernatremia and hyperchloremia. The Parkland/Baxter formula is used to calculate the volume of LR solution needed:

- 4 mL of LR X kg body weight X % TBSA burned (counting only full and partial thickness burns) = 24-hour volume.
- Example for 70 kg adult with 36% of TBSA burned: 4 x 70 X 36 = 10,080 mL.

Half of the volume is administered over the first 8 hours and the second half over the next 16 hours. So, using the example, the patient will receive 5040 mL in the first 8 hours at the rate of 630 mL/hr (5040/8); and in the next 16 hours, the patient will receive 315 ml/hr (5040/16). Fluid intake should be sufficient to produce 30 to 50 mL urine/hr. In the second 24 hours, fluid volume should be 1.5 to 2 times normal maintenance values with crystalloid with appropriate electrolyte balance.

PERMISSIVE HYPOTENSION

Permissive hypotension procedures allow the systolic blood pressure to fall low enough to prevent or control hemorrhage while still high enough to maintain perfusion. With trauma patients, this means restricting fluid resuscitation when active bleeding is occurring. While protocols vary, permissive hypotension usually includes systolic blood pressure ≤ 80 mm Hg although this may vary. For example, permissive hypotension with systolic blood pressure maintained at 80-100 mg may be indicated when massive transfusion protocols are activated. Permissive hypotension helps decrease some of the adverse effects associated with rapid and high-dose fluid resuscitation (emboli, coagulopathy, and hypothermia). However, the patient does remain at risk of hypoperfusion and must be monitored carefully. Permissive hypotension is generally contraindicated with brain or spinal cord injury although studies are ongoing (and mostly conducted with animals), and some controversy remains about the use of permissive hypotension.

MASSIVE TRANSFUSION PROTOCOL

Indications for activation of **massive transfusion protocol** (MTP) include:

- Actual/anticipated use of ≥4 units of RBCs in less than 4 hours or ≥10 units in 24 hours (some may need up to 30 units in 8 hours).
- Uncontrolled bleeding.
- Hemodynamic instability despite initial management of bleeding and resuscitation efforts that should include avoiding hypothermia and use of excessive crystalloid.
- Allowing permissive hypotension to 80-100 systolic to help control bleeding. Autotransfusion may be used when appropriate.

Protocols may vary somewhat:

- Activate based on criteria.
- Obtain baseline laboratory tests (CBC, coagulation screen, blood gases, and chemistry panel) and repeat CBC, blood gases, coagulation screen, and ionized calcium test every 30 to 60 minutes.
- Make request: Blood bank releases MTP pack, which varies but may contain 4 units PRBCs, 4 units FFP, and 1 unit (6-pack) platelets.
- If bleeding is controlled, MTP is discontinued, more packs are released (usually every 20 minutes or as needed).
- Targets include: Temperature >35° C, pH >7.2, base excess < -6, lactate <4 mmol/L, calcium >1.1 mmol/L, platelets >50,000, PT/APTT <1.5 times normal, INR ≤1.5, and fibrinogen ≥1.0 g/L.

ICP AND MONROE-KELLIE HYPOTHESIS

Increasing **intracranial pressure (ICP)** is a frequent complication of brain injuries, tumors, or other disorders affecting the brain, so monitoring the ICP is very important. Increased ICP can indicate cerebral edema, hemorrhage, and/or obstruction of cerebrospinal fluid. The Monroe-Kellie hypothesis states that in order to maintain a normal ICP, a change in volume in one compartment must be compensated by a reciprocal change in volume in another compartment. There are 3 compartments in the brain: the brain tissue, cerebrospinal fluid (CSF), and blood. The CSF and blood can change more easily to accommodate changes in pressure than tissue, so medical intervention focuses on cerebral blood flow and drainage. Normal ICP is 0-15 mm Hg on transducer or 80-180 mm H_2O on manometer. As intracranial pressure increases, **symptoms** include:

- Headache.
- Alterations in level of consciousness.
- Restlessness.
- Slowly reacting or nonreacting dilated or pinpoint pupils.
- Seizures.
- Motor weakness.
- Cushing's triad (late sign):
  o Increased systolic pressure with widened pulse pressure.
  o Bradycardia in response to increased pressure.
  o Decreased respirations.

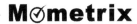

ICP Monitoring Devices

The **intracranial pressure (ICP) monitoring device** may be placed during surgery or a ventriculostomy performed in which a burr hole is drilled into the frontal area of the scalp and an **intraventricular catheter** threaded into the lateral ventricle. The intraventricular catheter may be used to monitor ICP and to drain excess CSF. Other monitoring devices include:

- **Intracranial pressure monitor bolt** (subarachnoid bolt) is applied through a burr hole with the distal end of the monitor probe resting in the subarachnoid space.
- **Epidural monitors** are placed into the epidural space.
- **Fiberoptic monitors** may be placed inside the brain.

The intraventricular catheter is the most accurate. CSF may be drained continuously or intermittently and must be monitored hourly for amount, color, and character. For ICP measurement, the patient's head must be elevated to 30 to 45° and the transducer leveled to the tragus of the ear or outer canthus of the eye, depending on facility policy. Normal ICP is 0-15 mm Hg on transducer or 80-180 mm H_2O on manometer.

Cerebral Blood Flow, MAP, and CPP

Mean arterial pressure (MAP) can be calculated as diastolic BP (DBP) + 1/3 pulse pressure. MAP has a direct effect on cerebral blood flow:

- Normal: 50 to 150 mm Hg.
- <50 mm Hg: Cerebral flow decreases, resulting in ischemia.
- >60 mm Hg: Needed to perfuse coronary arteries.
- 70 to 90 mm Hg: Needed to perfuse brains and other organs.
- 90 to 110 mm Hg needed to increase cerebral perfusion after neurosurgical procedures.
- >150 mm Hg: Cerebral blood vessels become maximally constricted and the brain barrier is disrupted, resulting in cerebral edema and increased ICP.

Cerebral perfusion pressure (CPP) is the pressure required to maintain adequate blood flow to the brain. CPP is based on mean arterial pressure (MAP), intracranial pressure (ICP), and jugular venous pressure (JVP). CPP is calculated as MAP - ICP (when ICP >JVP) OR MAP – JVP (when JVP > ICP):

- Normal: 60 to 100 mm Hg.
- <100 mm Hg: Hyperperfusion occurs with increased ICP.
- <60 mm Hg: Hypoperfusion occurs with ischemia.
- <30 mm Hg: Hypoperfusion is marked and incompatible with life.

Thermoregulation in Critically Ill Patients

The hypothalamus, limbic system, lower brainstem, reticular formation, spinal cord and sympathetic ganglia all play a role in regulation of core temperature. The normal core body temperature of 35.5-37.5 degrees Celsius is a narrow range which is frequently disrupted in the critically ill patient. **Impaired thermoregulation** can occur in patients with sepsis, brain or spinal cord trauma, stroke, and tumors of the central nervous system. Mild hypothermia is common during deep sedation. Hypothermia (core temperature of <35 degrees Celsius) is associated with an increased risk of post-operative wound infections, blood loss and adverse cardiovascular events. Hypothermia may occur in trauma patients, patients with sepsis, post-operative patients and patients with severe burns. Hyperthermia (core temperature of >38 degrees Celsius) may occur in systemic inflammatory response syndrome, malignant hyperthermia, heat stroke, neuroleptic malignant syndrome, and serotonin syndrome. Hyperpyrexia

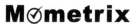

occurs when the core temperature exceeds 40 degrees Celsius. Core temperatures exceeding 41.5 degrees Celsius may be life-threatening.

THERAPEUTIC HYPOTHERMIA

Therapeutic hypothermia is used to reduce ischemic tissue damage associated with cardiac arrest, ischemic stroke, traumatic brain/spinal cord injury, neurogenic fever, and subsequent coma (3 on Glasgow scale). Hypothermia has a neuroprotective effect by making cell membranes less permeable, thus reducing neurologic edema and damage. Hypothermia should be initiated immediately after an ischemic event if possible but some benefit remains up to 6 hours. Hypothermia to 33°C may be induced by cooled saline through a femoral catheter, reducing temperature 1.5 to 2° C per hour, with by an electronic control unit. Hypothermic water blankets covering ≥80% of body the body surface can also lower body temperature. In some cases, both a femoral cooling catheter and water blanket are used for rapid reduction of temperature. Rectal probes are used to measure core temperature, but Foley temperature catheters are more common. Desflurane or meperidine is given to reduce the shivering response. Hypothermia increases risk of bleeding (decreased clotting time), infection (due to impairing leukocyte function and introducing catheters), arrhythmias, hyperglycemia, and DVT. Rewarming is done slowly at 0.5 to 1° C/hr. through warmed intravenous fluids, warm humidified air, and/or warming blanket. The warming process is a critical time as it causes potassium to be moved from extracellular to intracellular spaces and the patient's electrolyte levels must be monitored regularly.

HEMODYNAMIC MONITORING AND OXYGEN SATURATION

Hemodynamic monitoring includes monitoring **oxygen saturation** levels, which must be maintained for proper cardiac function. The central venous catheter often has an oxygen sensor at the tip to monitor oxygen saturation in the right atrium. If the catheter tip is located near the renal veins, this can cause an increase in right atrial oxygen saturation; and near the coronary sinus, a decrease.

- Increased oxygen saturation may result from left atrial to right atrial shunt, abnormal pulmonary venous return, increased delivery of oxygen or decrease in extraction of oxygen.
- Decreased oxygen saturation may be related to low cardiac output with an increase in oxygen extraction or decrease in arterial oxygen saturation with normal differences in the atrial and ventricular oxygen saturation.

MINIMALLY/NON-INVASIVE HEMODYNAMIC MONITORING

Hemodynamic monitoring and evaluation of cardiac function is an important component of the care of the critically ill patient. **Minimally or non-invasive** alternatives to traditional invasive means of hemodynamic monitoring (such as the use of a pulmonary artery catheter) include esophageal Doppler, arterial pressure based cardiac output monitoring, and impedance cardiography. Esophageal Doppler is a minimally invasive option used in surgical patients to monitor descending aortic blood flow and estimate cardiac output. A probe is inserted into the esophagus and then connected to a monitor, where waveform shapes produced by aortic blood flow are displayed.

Arterial pressure based cardiac output monitors (APCO's) use an algorithm to estimate cardiac output through the analysis of the arterial pressure waveform. The radial or femoral artery is accessed using a standard arterial catheter and no external calibration is needed.

Impedance cardiography is a non-invasive method of hemodynamic monitoring in which sensors placed on the body use electrical signals to measure the level of change in impedance in the thoracic fluid. A waveform is generated and is then used to calculate cardiac output and stroke volume, as well as ten additional hemodynamic parameters.

INTRAARTERIAL BLOOD PRESSURE MONITORING

Intraarterial blood pressure monitoring uses a catheter to measure systolic, diastolic, and mean arterial pressures (MAP) continuously. Before catheter insertion, collateral circulation must be assessed by Doppler or the Allen test (radial). Complications include arterial vasospasm, hematoma formation, hemorrhage (accidental disconnect), catheter occlusion, compartment syndrome, retroperitoneal bleed (femoral site), and thrombus/embolus.

- **Set up:** The line should be connected to the monitor and a pressure bag set at 300mHg with no longer than 3 feet of stiff, noncompliant tubing to ensure accuracy. The transducer is leveled at the phlebostatic axis of the patient. The line should be kept free of any air or bubbles, and re-zeroed every four hours and with a change of patient position.
- **Waveform:** A normal ABP waveform should be smooth and regular, with a dicrotic notch. To test, perform a "square-wave" or "Fast Flush" test; flush the line while watching the monitor. There should be a square shape, followed by two oscillations and a return to normal waves. A missing dicrotic notch indicates a blockage of some kind (thrombus, plaque, and vasospasm) or low pressure in the bag. Too many oscillations or an increased sharpness of the wave indicates under dampening and is caused by increased SVR or too long of tubing.

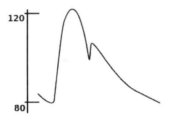

FIBRINOLYTIC INFUSIONS

Fibrinolytic infusion is indicated for acute myocardial infarction under these conditions:

- Symptoms of MI, <6-12 hours since onset of symptoms.
- ≥1 mm elevation of ST in ≥2 contiguous leads.
- No contraindications and no cardiogenic shock.

Fibrinolytic agents should be administered as soon as possible, within 30 minutes is best. All agents convert plasminogen to plasmin, which breaks down fibrin, dissolving clots:

- Streptokinase & anistreplase (1st generation).
- Alteplase or tissue plasminogen activator (tPA) (second generation).
- Reteplase & tenecteplase (3rd generation).

Relative contraindications include: Active peptic ulcer, >10 minutes of CPR, advanced renal or hepatic disease, pregnancy, anticoagulation therapy, acute uncontrolled hypertension/chronic poorly controlled hypertension, recent (2-4 weeks) internal bleeding, noncompressible vascular punctures.

Absolute contraindications include: Present or recent bleeding or history of severe bleeding, history of intracranial hemorrhage, history of stroke (<3 months unless within 3 hours), aortic dissection, pericarditis, intracranial/ intraspinal surgery or trauma within 3 months, neoplasm, aneurysm, or AVM.

THROMBOLYTICS

Thrombolytics are drugs used to dissolve clots in myocardial infarction, ischemic stroke, DVT, and pulmonary embolism. Thrombolytics may be given in combination with heparin or low-weight heparin to increase anticoagulation effect. Thrombolytics should be administered within 90 minutes but may be given up to 6 hours after an event. They may increase the danger of hemorrhage and are contraindicated with hemorrhagic strokes, recent surgery, or bleeding. Thrombolytics include:

- **Alteplase tissue-type plasminogen activator** (t-PA) (Activase®) is an enzyme that converts plasminogen to plasmin, which is a fibrinolytic enzyme. T-PA is used for ischemic stroke, MI, and pulmonary embolism and must be given IV within 3-4.5 hours or by catheter directly to the site of occlusion within 6 hours.
- **Anistreplase** (Eminase®) is used for treatment of acute MI and is given intravenously in a 30-unit dose over 2-5 minutes.
- **Reteplase** (Retavase®) is a plasminogen activator used after MI to prevent CHF (contraindicated for ischemic strokes). It is given in 2 doses, a 10-unit bolus over 2 minutes and then repeated in 30 minutes.
- **Streptokinase** (Streptase®) is used for pulmonary emboli, acute MI, intracoronary thrombi, DVT, and arterial thromboembolism. It should be given within 4 hours but can be given up to 24 hours. Intravenous infusion is usually 1,500,000 units in 60 minutes. Intracoronary infusion is done with an initial 20,000-unit bolus and then 2000 units per minute for 60 minutes.
- **Tenecteplase** (TNKase®) is used to treat acute MI with large ST elevation. It is administered in a one-time bolus over 5 seconds and should be administered within 30 minutes of event.

Contraindications to thrombolytic therapy include:

- Evidence of cerebral or subarachnoid hemorrhage or other internal bleeding or history of intracranial hemorrhage, recent stroke, head trauma, or surgery. Ruled out by CT scan before administration for ischemic stroke.
- Uncontrolled hypertension, seizures.
- Intracranial AVM, neoplasm, or aneurysm.
- Current anticoagulation therapy.
- Low platelet count (<100,000 mm³).

HSS

Hypertonic saline solution (HSS) has a sodium concentration higher than 0.9% (NS) and is used to reduce intracranial pressure/cerebral edema and treat traumatic brain injury. Concentrations usually range from 2% to 23.4%. The hypertonic solution draws fluid from the tissue through osmosis. As edema decreases, circulation improves. HSS also expands plasma, increasing CPP, and counteracts hyponatremia that occurs in the brain after injury. Administration:

- Peripheral lines: HSS <3% only.
- Central lines: HSS ≥3%

HSS can be administered continuously at rates varying from 30 mL to 150 mL/hr. Rate must be carefully controlled. Fluid status must be monitored to prevent hypovolemia, which increases risk of renal failure. Boluses (typically 30 mL of 23.4%) may be administered over 15 minutes for acute increased ICP or transtentorial herniation. Laboratory monitoring includes:

- Sodium (every 6 hours): Maintain at 145 to 155 mmol/L. Higher levels can cause heart/respiratory/renal failure.
- Serum osmolality (every 12 hours): Maintain at 320 mOsmol/L. Hgher levels can cause renal failure.

MANNITOL

Mannitol is an osmotic diuretic that increases excretion of both sodium and water and reduces intracranial pressure and brain mass, especially after traumatic brain injury. Mannitol may also be used to shrink the cells of the blood-brain barrier in order to help other medications breach this barrier. Mannitol is administered per intravenous infusion:

- 0.25g to 2g/kg in a 15% to 25% solution over one-half to one hour.

Cerebral spinal fluid pressure should show decrease within 15 minutes. Fluid and electrolyte balances must be carefully monitored as well as I &O and body weight. Concentrations of 20% to 25% require a filter. Crystals may form if the mannitol solution is too cold and the mannitol container may require heating (in 80° C water) and shaking to dissolve crystals, but solution should be cooled to ≤body temperature prior to administration. Mannitol cannot be administered in polyvinylchloride bags as precipitates form. Side effects include fluid and electrolyte imbalance, nausea, vomiting, hypotension, tachycardia, fever, and urticaria.

PHARMACOLOGIC MEASURES MAXIMIZING PERFUSION IN PERIPHERALY VASCULAR DISEASE

The primary focus of pharmacologic measures to ma**ximize perfusion in peripheral vascular disease** is to reduce the risk of thromboses/acute vascular occlusion:

- **Antiplatelet agents**, such as aspirin, Ticlid®, and Plavix®, which interfere with the function of the plasma membrane, reducing clotting of the blood. These agents are ineffective to treat clots but prevent clot formation.
- **Vasodilators** may divert blood from already ischemic areas, but some may be indicated, such as Pletal®, which dilates arteries and decreases clotting, and is used for control of intermittent claudication.
- **Antilipemic,** such as Zocor® and Questran®, slow progression of atherosclerosis.
- **Hemorrheologics,** such as Trental®, reduce fibrinogen, reducing blood viscosity and rigidity of erythrocytes; however, clinical studies show limited benefit. It may be used for intermittent claudication.
- **Analgesics** may be necessary to improve quality of life. Opioids may be needed in some cases.
- **Thrombolytics** may be injected into a blocked artery under angiography to dissolve clots.
- **Anticoagulants**, such as Coumadin® and Lovenox®, prevent blood clots from forming.

MEDICATIONS FOR HEART FAILURE

- **ACE inhibitors:** Captopril (Capoten®), enalapril (Vasotec®), and lisinopril (Prinivil®): Decrease afterload/preload and reverse ventricular remodeling; also prevent neuropathy in DM. Contraindicated with renal insufficiency, renal artery stenosis, and pregnancy.
  - Side effects include cough (#1), hyperkalemia, hypotension, angioedema, dizziness, and weakness.

- **Angiotensin receptor blockers (ARBs):** Losartan (Cozaar®) and valsartan (Diovan®): Decrease afterload/preload and reverse ventricular remodeling, causing vasodilation and reducing blood pressure. They are used for those who cannot tolerate ACE inhibitors.
  - Side effects include cough (less common than with ACE inhibitors), hyperkalemia, hypotension, headache, dizziness, metallic taste, and rash.

- **β-Blockers:** Metoprolol (Lopressor®), carvedilol (Coreg®) and esmolol (Brevibloc®) Slow the heart rate, reduce hypertension, prevent dysrhythmias, and reverse ventricular remodeling. Contraindicated in bradyarrythmias, decompensated HF, uncontrolled hypoglycemia/ diabetes mellitus, and airway disease.

- o   Side effects: bradycardia, hypotension, bronchospasm, may mask signs of hypoglycemia.
- **Aldosterone antagonists: Spironolactone (Aldactone®):** Decreases preload and myocardial hypertrophy and reduces edema and sodium retention but may increase serum potassium.
- **Furosemide (Lasix®)** is used for the control of congestive heart failure as well as renal insufficiency. It is used after surgery to decrease preload and to reduce the inflammatory response caused by cardiopulmonary bypass (post-perfusion syndrome).

SMOOTH MUSCLE RELAXANTS AND CALCIUM CHANNEL BLOCKERS

Smooth muscle relaxants:

- Decrease peripheral vascular resistance; may cause hypotension and headaches.
- Sodium nitroprusside (Nipride®) dilates both arteries and veins; rapid-acting and used for reduction of hypertension and afterload reduction for heart failure.
- Nitroglycerin (Tridil®) primarily dilates veins and is used sublingual or IV to reduce preload for acute heart failure, unstable angina, and acute MI. Nitroglycerin may also be used prophylactically after PCIs to prevent vasospasm.
- Hydralazine (Apresoline®) dilates arteries and is given intermittently to reduce hypertension.

Calcium Channel blockers:

- Primarily arterial vasodilators that may affect the peripheral and/or coronary arteries.
- Side effects: lethargy, flushing, edema, ascites, and indigestion:
- Nifedipine (Procardia®) and nicardipine (Cardene®) are primarily arterial vasodilators, used to treat acute hypertension. Diltiazem (Cardizem®) and Verapamil (Calan®, Isoptin®) dilate primarily coronary arteries and slow the heart rate, thus are used for angina, atrial fibrillation, and SVT. *Note:* Nifedipine (Procardia®) should be avoided in older adults due to increased risk of hypotension and myocardial ischemia.

B-TYPE NATRIURETIC PEPTIDES, ALPHA-ADRENERGIC BLOCKERS, AND SELECTIVE SPECIFIC DOPAMINE DA-1 RECEPTOR AGONISTS

B-type natriuretic peptide (BNP) (Nesiritide—Natrecor®):

- A type of vasodilator (non-inotropic), which is a recombinant form of a peptide of the human brain.
- It decreases filling pressure, vascular resistance, and increases U/O.
- May cause hypotension, headache, bradycardia, and nausea. It is used short term for worsening decompensated CHF; contraindicated in SBP<90, cardiogenic shock, contrictive pericarditis, or valve stenosis.

Alpha-adrenergic blockers:

- Block alpha receptors in arteries and veins, causing vasodilation
- May cause orthostatic hypotension and edema from fluid retention:
- Labetalol (Normodyne®) is a combination peripheral alpha-blocker and cardiac β-blocker and is used to treat acute hypertension, acute stroke, and acute aortic dissection. Phentolamine (Regitine®) is a peripheral arterial dilator that reduces afterload. It is used for HTN crisis in patients with pheochromocytoma, as well as a subcutaneous injection for extravasation of vessicants.

Selective specific dopamine DA-1-receptor agonists:

- Fenoldopam (Corlopam®):A peripheral dilator affecting renal and mesenteric arteries and can be used for patients with renal dysfunction or those at risk of renal insufficiency.

INOTROPIC AGENTS

Inotropic agents are drugs used to increase cardiac output and improve contractibility. IV inotropic agents may increase the risk of death, but may be used when other drugs fail. Oral forms of these drugs are less effective than intravenous. Inotropic agents include:

- **β-Adrenergic agonists:**
  - *Dobutamine* improves cardiac output, treats cardiac decompensation, and increases blood pressure. It helps the body to utilize norepinephrine. Side effects include increased or labile blood pressure, increased heart rate, PVCs, N/V, and bronchospasm.
  - *Dopamine* improves cardiac output, blood pressure, and blood flow to the renal and mesenteric arteries. Side effects include tachycardia or bradycardia, palpitations, BP changes, dyspnea, nausea and vomiting, headache, and gangrene of extremities.
- **Phosphodiesterase III inhibitors:**
  - *Milrinone* (Primacor®) increases strength of contractions and cause vasodilation. Side effects include ventricular arrhythmias, hypotension, and headaches.
- **Digoxin (Lanoxin®):**
  - Increases contractibility and cardiac output and prevents arrhythmias.

LOOP DIURETICS

Diuretics increase renal perfusion and filtration, thereby reducing preload and decreasing peripheral and pulmonary edema, hypertension, CHF, diabetes insipidus, and osteoporosis. There are different types of diuretics: loop, thiazide, and potassium sparing. **Loop diuretics** inhibit the reabsorption of sodium and chloride (primarily) in the ascending loop of Henle. They also cause increased secretion of other electrolytes, such as calcium, magnesium, and potassium, and this can result in imbalances that cause dysrhythmias. Other side effects include frequent urination, postural hypotension, and increased blood sugar and uric acid levels. They are short-acting so are less effective than other diuretics for control of hypertension:

- **Bumetanide** (Bumex®) is given intravenously after surgery to reduce preload or orally to treat heart failure.
- **Ethacrynic acid** (Edecrin®) is given intravenously after surgery to reduce preload.
- **Furosemide** (Lasix®) is used for the control of congestive heart failure as well as renal insufficiency. It is used after surgery to decrease preload and to reduce the inflammatory response caused by cardiopulmonary bypass (post-perfusion syndrome).

THIAZIDE DIURETICS

Thiazide diuretics inhibit the reabsorption of sodium and chloride primarily in the early distal tubules, forcing more sodium and water to be excreted. Thiazide diuretics increase secretion of potassium and bicarbonate, so they are often given with supplementary potassium or in combination with potassium-sparing diuretics. They have a long duration of action (12-72 hours, depending on the drug) so they are able to maintain control of hypertension better than short-acting drugs. They may be given daily or 3-5 days per week. There are numerous thiazide diuretics, including:

- Chlorothiazide (Diuril®)
- Bendroflumethiazide (Naturetin®)

- Chlorthalidone (Hygroton®)
- Trichlormethiazide (Naqua®)

Side effects include, dizziness, lightheadedness, postural hypotension, headache, blurred vision, and itching, especially during initial treatment. Thiazide diuretics cause sensitivity to sun exposure, so people should be counseled to use sunscreen.

POTASSIUM-SPARING DIURETICS

Potassium-sparing diuretics inhibit the reabsorption of sodium in the late distal tubule and collecting duct. They are weaker than thiazide or loop diuretics, but do not cause a reduction in potassium level; however, if used alone, they may cause an increase in potassium, which can cause weakness, irregular pulse, and cardiac arrest. Because potassium-sparing diuretics are less effective alone, they are often given in a combined form with a thiazide diuretic (usually chlorothiazide), which mitigates the potassium imbalance. Typical side effects include dehydration, blurred vision, nausea insomnia, and nasal congestion, especially in the first few days of treatment:

- **Spironolactone** (Aldactone®) is a synthetic steroid diuretic that increases the secretion of both water and sodium and is used to treat congestive heart failure. It may be given orally or intravenously.
- **Eplerenone** is an antimineralocorticoid similar to spironolactone but with fewer side effects.

ANTICOAGULANTS

Anticoagulants are used to prevent thrombo-emboli. All pose risk of bleeding:

- **Aspirin:** Often used prophylactically to prevent clots and poses less danger of bleeding than other drugs. Do not give to adolescents (risk of Reyes syndrome).
- **Warfarin (Coumadin®):** Blocks utilization of vitamin K and decreases production of clotting factors. Oral medications for those at risk of developing blood clots, such as those with mechanical heart valves, atrial fibrillation, and clotting disorders. Antidote: Vitamin K.
- **Heparin:** The primary intravenous anticoagulant and increases the activity of antithrombin III. It is used for those with MI and those undergoing PCI or other cardiac surgery, as well as patients with active clots. Monitored by aPTT or AntiXa; monitor for signs of heparin-induced thrombocytopenia (HIT)- an allergic response to heparin that causes a platelet count drop <150,000, usually to 30-50% of baseline, usually occurring 5-14 days after beginning heparin.
- **Dalteparin (Fragmin®) & Enoxaparin (Lovenox®):** Low-molecular weight heparins that increase activity of antithrombin III used for DVT prophylaxis, unstable angina, MI, and cardiac surgery.
- **Bivalirudin (Angiomax®):** Direct thrombin inhibitors used for unstable angina, PCI, and for prophylaxis and treatment of thrombosis in heparin-induced thrombocytopenia (HIT).

NEUROMUSCULAR BLOCKADE

Neuromuscular blockades relax muscles for surgical procedures, aid in intubation, reduce extreme agitation and skeletal muscle activity, facilitate mechanical ventilation, and prevent increased ICP with intracranial hypertension. Sedatives/analgesics should be given prior to and during neuromuscular blockade to prevent PTSD from recall of pain. Neuromuscular blocking agents (NMBA) may cause muscle weakness, myopathy, and bronchoconstriction from release of histamine. Apnea and airway obstruction may occur:

- **Depolarizing agents** (agonists), such as succinylcholine, bind directly to acetylcholine receptors, blocking access and activating the receptor to depolarize. Some drugs potentiate effects: Numerous antibiotics (streptomycin, tetracycline, and clindamycin), antiarrhythmics (quinidine, CCBs), lithium carbonate, and magnesium sulfate. Side effects include myalgia, malignant hyperthermia, and severe anaphylactic/anaphylactoid reactions.
- **Non-depolarizing agents** (antagonists) bind directly to acetylcholine receptors, blocking access, but do not activate the receptors, so depolarization does not occur. Non-depolarizing agents are further classified by duration of action: short acting (mivacurium, rapacuronium), intermediate acting (rocuronium, vecuronium, atracurium, cisatracurium), and long acting (pancuronium, doxacurium, pipecuronium). Non-depolarizing NMBAs have slower onset and longer duration than succinylcholine.

ANTICONVULSANTS
Anticonvulsants:

- **Primidone** (Mysoline®) - Use: Grand mal, psychomotor, and focal seizures. Side Effects: double vision, ataxia, impotence, lethargy, and irritability. Toxic reactions include skin rash.
- **Tiagabine** (Gabitril®) - Use: Partial seizures. Side Effects: Concentration problems, weak knees, dysarthria, abdominal pain, tremor, dizziness, fatigue, and agitation.
- **Topiramate** (Topamax®) - Use: Partial and tonic-clonic seizures, migraines. Side Effects: anorexia, weight loss, somnolence, ataxia, and confusion. Toxic reactions include kidney stones.
- **Valproate/Valproic acid** (Depakote®, Depakene®) – Use: Complex partial, simple, and complex absence seizures. Bipolar disorder. Side Effects: weight gain, alopecia, tremor, menstrual disorders, nausea, and vomiting. Toxic reactions include hepatotoxicity, severe pancreatitis, rash, blood dyscrasias, and nephritis.
- **Zonisamide** (Zonegran®, Excegran®) – Use: Partial seizures. Side Effects: Anorexia, nausea, agitation, rash, headache, dizziness, and somnolence. Toxic reactions include leukopenia and hepatotoxicity.
- **Carbamazepine** (Tegretol®) - Use: Partial, tonic-clonic, and absence seizures. Analgesia for trigeminal neuralgia. Side effects: Dizziness, drowsiness, nausea, and vomiting. Toxic reactions include severe skin rash, agranulocytosis, aplastic anemia, and hepatitis
- **Clonazepam** (Klonopin®) - Use: Akinetic, absence, and myoclonic seizures. Lennox-Gastaut syndrome. Side effects: Behavioral changes, hirsutism or alopecia, headaches, and drowsiness. Toxic reactions include hepatotoxicity, thrombocytopenia, ataxia, and bone marrow failure.
- **Ethosuximide** (Zarontin®) -Use: Absence seizures. Side effects: Headaches and gastrointestinal disorders. Toxic reactions include skin rash, blood dyscrasias (sometimes fatal), hepatitis and lupus erythematosus.
- **Felbamate** (Felbatol®) - Use: Lennox-Gastaut syndrome. Side effects: Headache, fatigue, insomnia, and cognitive impairment. Toxic reactions include aplastic anemia and hepatic failure. It is recommended only if other medications have failed.
- **Fosphenytoin** (Cerebyx®) - Use: Status epilepticus. Prevention and treatment during neurosurgery. Side effects: CNS depression, hypotension, cardiovascular collapse, dizziness, nystagmus, pruritus.
- **Gabapentin** (Neurontin®) - Use: Partial seizures, diabetic neuropathy. Side effects: Post-herpetic neuralgia. Dizziness, somnolence, drowsiness, ataxia, weight gain, and nausea. Toxic reactions include hepatotoxicity and leukopenia.

- **Lamotrigine** (Lamictal®) - Use: Partial and primary generalized tonic-clonic seizures. - Lennox-Gastaut syndrome. Side effects: Tremor, ataxia, weight gain, dizziness, headache, and drowsiness. Toxic reactions include severe rash, which may require hospitalization.
- **Levetiracetam** (Keppra®) - Use: Partial onset, myoclonic, and generalized tonic-clonic seizures. Side effects: Idiopathic generalized epilepsy, dizziness, somnolence, irritability, alopecia, double vision, sore throat, and fatigue. Toxic reactions include bone marrow suppression and liver failure.
- **Oxcarbazepine** (Trileptal®) - Use: Partal seizures. Side effects- Double or abnormal vision, tremor, abnormal gait, GI disorders, dizziness, and fatigue. A toxic reaction is hepatotoxicity.
- **Phenobarbital** (Luminal®) - Use: Tonic-clonic and cortical local seizures. Acute convulsive episodes. Hypnotic for insomnia. Side effects: Sedation, double vision, agitation, and ataxia. Toxic reactions include anemia and skin rash.
- **Phenytoin** (Dilantin®) -Use: Tonic-clonic and complex partial seizures. Side effects: Nystagmus, vision disorders, gingival hyperplasia, hirsutism, dysrhythmias, and dysarthria. Toxic reactions include collapse of cardiovascular system and CNS depression

EPINEPHRINE TO TREAT ANAPHYLAXIS

Anaphylaxis is a severe, systemic hypersensitivity (allergic) reaction that is classified as a type I hypersensitivity. If an individual suffering from an anaphylactic reaction is not treated immediately, death is likely. The systemic symptoms of anaphylaxis (hypotension, difficulty breathing, and angioedema) result from the release of large amounts of histamine from mast cells. When released into the bloodstream, histamine causes the bronchioles to constrict; it also causes vasodilation (relaxation of the blood vessels, resulting in a decrease in blood pressure) and leakage of fluids into the surrounding tissue (resulting in edema and a further decline in blood pressure). When an individual is suffering from an anaphylactic reaction, treatment with epinephrine is the best way to stabilize the patient. **Epinephrine** is a powerful vasoconstrictor, and an equally powerful bronchodilator. It also increases heart rate and stroke volume to counteract the shock that occurs as a result of the anaphylactic reaction.

PHARMACOLOGIC TREATMENT OF WOUND PAIN

TOPICAL ANESTHETICS

There are numerous different types of pain medications that may be used to control pain from wounds, including **topical anesthetics**:

- **Lidocaine 2-4%** is frequently used during debridement or dressing changes. Lidocaine is useful only superficially and may take 15-30 minutes before it is effective.
- **Eutectic Mixture of Local Anesthetics (EMLA Cream)** provides good pain control. The wound is first cleansed and then the cream is applied thickly (1/4 inch) extending about 1/2 inch past the wound to the peri-wound tissue. The wound is then covered with plastic wrap, which is secured and left in place for about 20 minutes. The wrapped time may be extended to 45-60 minute if necessary to completely numb the tissue. The tissue should remain numb for about 1 hour after the plastic wrap is removed, allowing time for the wound to be cleansed, debrided, and/or redressed.

REGIONAL ANESTHESIA

Regional anesthesia (injectable subcutaneous and perineural medications) is used administered locally about the wound or as nerve blocks. Medications include lidocaine, bupivacaine and tetracaine in solution. Epinephrine is sometimes added to increase vasoconstriction and reduce bleeding although it is avoided in distal areas of the limbs (hands and feet) to prevent ischemia.

- **Field blockade** involves injecting the anesthetic into the periwound tissue or into the wound margins. The effect may be decreased by inflammation. The effects last for limited periods of time.
- **Regional nerve blocks** may involve single injections, the effects of which are limited in duration but can provide pain relief for treatments. Techniques that use continuous catheter infusions are longer lasting and can be controlled more precisely. Blocks may involve nerves proximal to affected areas, such as peripheral nerve blocks, or large nerve blocks near the spinal cord, such as percutaneous lumbar sympathetic blocks (LSB). Long-term blocks may use alcohol-based medications to permanently inactivate the nerves.

SYSTEMIC MEDICATIONS

Systemic medications may be given orally or by injection into muscles, subcutaneous tissue, or veins. The 3-step World Health Organization (WHO) "Analgesic Ladder" is frequently used as a point of reference. Combinations of drugs are often more effective than one alone:

- **Step 1**: Mild to moderate pain is treated with aspirin, acetaminophen, and NSAIDs.
- **Step 2:** Moderate to severe pain unrelieved by Step 1 medications may need opioids, such as codeine, tramadol, or Percocet®.
- **Step 3:** Severe pain without relief from Step 1 or Step 2 medications may need stronger opioids, such as morphine, Dilaudid®, or MS-Contin®.

Note: Meperidine (Demerol®) should not be used for pain control because prolonged use may result in dependence, high doses may cause seizures, and a metabolite of meperidine (normeperidine) may accumulate. It is short acting and peaks quickly but may be indicated for occasional use.

SEDATION
PROPOFOL

Sedation used for drug-induced coma often includes **propofol**. Propofol is an IV non-opioid hypnotic anesthetic, the most common used for induction. It is also used for maintenance and postoperative sedation. Onset of action is rapid because of high lipid solubility, and propofol has a short distribution half-life and rapid clearance, so recovery is also fast. Propofol is metabolized by the liver as well as through the lungs. Propofol decreases cerebral blood flow, metabolic rate of oxygen consumption and ICP. Propofol causes vasodilation with resultant hypotension, but with bradycardia rather than tachycardia. Propofol is a respiratory depressant, resulting in apnea after induction and decreased tidal volume, respiratory rate, and hypoxic drive during maintenance. Propofol has antiemetic properties as well but does not produce analgesia.

CONSCIOUS SEDATION

Conscious sedation is used to decrease sensations of pain and awareness caused by a surgical or invasive procedure, such a biopsy, chest tube insertion, fracture repair, and endoscopy. It is also used during presurgical preparations, such as insertion of central lines, catheters, and use of cooling blankets. Conscious sedation uses a combination of analgesia and sedation so that patients can remain responsive and follow verbal cues but have a brief amnesia preventing recall of the procedures. The patient must be monitored carefully, including pulse oximetry, during this type of sedation. The most commonly used drugs include:

- **Midazolam** (Versed®): This is a short-acting water-soluble sedative, with onset of 1-5 minutes, peaking in 30, and duration usually about 1 hour (but may last up to 6 hours).
- **Fentanyl**: This is a short-acting opioid with immediate onset, peaking in 10-15 minutes and with duration of about 20-45 minutes.

The fentanyl/midazolam combination provides both sedation and pain control. Conscious sedation usually requires 6 hours fasting prior to administration.

BARBITURATES

Sedation may be used for drug-induced coma to treat traumatic brain injury and increased intracranial pressure. The most commonly used drugs are barbiturates (pentobarbital or thiopental) and sedatives (propofol). **Barbiturates** depress the reticular activating system in the brain stem, an area controlling body functions, including consciousness. Barbiturates with phenyl serve as anticonvulsants (phenobarbital) but those with methyl (methohexital) do not. If sulfur is added to the compound to replace some oxygen, the barbiturates have increased lipid solubility (thiopental, methohexital, and thiamylal), making them useful as rapid acting anesthetics. Barbiturates have a number of systemic effects. Blood pressure falls and heart rate increases although cardiac output is usually maintained. With hypovolemia, CHF, and β-adrenergic blockade, there may be peripheral pooling of blood and myocardial depression that causes a pronounced drop in BP and cardiac output. Barbiturates reduce cerebral blood flow and decrease ICP, but cerebral oxygen consumption is also reduced. Barbiturates do not relax muscles or reduce sensation of pain.

MECHANICAL VENTILATION

Patients intubated for mechanical ventilation are usually given **sedation and/or analgesia** initially, but medications should be reduced and given in boluses rather than with continuous IV drip with a goal of stopping sedation as it prolongs ventilation time. Typical sedatives include midazolam, propofol, and lorazepam. Narcotic analgesics include fentanyl and morphine sulfate. Uses of sedation include:

- Controlling agitation and excessive movement that may interfere with ventilation.
- Reduce pain and discomfort associated with ventilation.
- Control respiratory distress.

Triglyceride levels must be checked periodically if propofol is administered for >24-48 hours. Neuromuscular blocking agents are rarely used because they may cause long-term weakness and increase length of ventilation although they may be indicated in some cases, such as with excessive shivering or cardiac arrest. Many patients are able to tolerate mechanical ventilation without sedation, and sedation should always be decreased to the minimal amount necessary as excess sedation may delay extubation.

Review Video: **Medical Ventilators**
Visit mometrix.com/academy and enter code: 679637

TCRN Practice Test

1. When monitoring intracranial pressure in an adult, the trauma nurse must be aware that normal range is

   a. 5 to 10 mm Hg.
   b. 10 to 15 mm Hg.
   c. 15 to 20 mm Hg.
   d. 20 to 25 mm Hg.

2. With a gunshot wound to the abdomen, the trauma nurse should anticipate that the organ most likely to be injured is the

   a. colon.
   b. stomach.
   c. liver.
   d. small intestine.

3. A 40-year old male receives mannitol to decrease increased intracranial pressure resulting from a traumatic brain injury and exhibits cardiac arrhythmias. Which of the following electrolyte abnormalities associated with mannitol administration is most likely the cause of the arrhythmias?

   a. Hyperkalemia.
   b. Hypokalemia.
   c. Hypernatremia
   d. Hypermagnesemia.

4. If a handgun is found in the pocket of a trauma victim, the first consideration when removing and securing the gun is to

   a. place it in a paper bag.
   b. arrange for security personnel to remove the gun.
   c. avoid touching the trigger.
   d. call the police.

5. If a patient with facial fractures has dentoalveolar trauma with avulsion of permanent teeth, reimplantation should ideally be carried out within

   a. 15 minutes.
   b. 30 minutes.
   c. 60 minutes.
   d. 120 minutes.

6. When utilizing the AMPLE acronym to rapidly obtain important information about the patient's history, the L stands for

   a. last meal.
   b. length of time since injury.
   c. legal directives.
   d. loss of blood.

7. An 11-month old boy climbed out of his highchair and fell onto a tile floor, hitting his head. At 48 hours he experienced a seizure and exhibited fever, weakness on the right side, poor feeding, and pronounced lethargy, indicating a subdural hematoma. Which emergent treatment is most indicated?

    a. Insertion of an intracranial pressure-monitoring device.
    b. Intravenous mannitol.
    c. Intravenous hypertonic saline solution.
    d. Surgical evacuation of hematoma.

8. During transport of a patient with depressed respirations from the scene of an accident to the trauma center, the oxygen delivery device that provides the highest level of FIO_2 is

    a. partial rebreather face mask.
    b. Venturi mask.
    c. non-rebreather mask.
    d. nasal cannula.

9. Which of the following patients is least likely to require intracranial pressure monitoring?

    a. Fifty-year old female with head injury, Glasgow coma score of 14, and BP of 95/60.
    b. Forty-five-year-old head injury patient with BP of 80/40 and unilateral posturing.
    c. Four-year old with extensive subarachnoid hemorrhage.
    d. Sixteen-year-old with acute head injury and unable to follow commands.

10. Which of the following is an absolute contraindication to nasotracheal intubation?

    a. Cervical spine injury
    b. Facial trauma.
    c. Skull fracture.
    d. Apnea.

11. With targeted temperature management (TTM), AKA therapeutic hypothermia, the patient's temperature should generally be lowered and maintained at

    a. 24 to 28° C.
    b. 28 to 30° C.
    c. 30 to 32° C.
    d. 32 to 36° C.

12. A colleague tells a newly-hired trauma nurse, "The suggestions you made were a complete waste of time, and if you want to get along with the staff you need to stop trying to make changes." This is an example of which of the following?

    a. Discrimination.
    b. Horizontal/Lateral violence.
    c. Advice.
    d. Vertical violence.

13. If the paramedic reports that a patient in transit has a Glasgow Coma Score of 7, the trauma nurse expects the patient to

    a. have had brief periods of loss of consciousness but to be alert and responsive.
    b. remain slightly confused but able to follow verbal direction.
    c. exhibit focal neurological defects.
    d. be intubated and comatose.

14. The primary purpose of using rapid sequence intubation (RSI) is to:

    a. reduce the risk of gastric aspiration.
    b. prevent esophageal trauma.
    c. speed intubation.
    d. reduce tracheal trauma.

15. If a burn patient's fluid resuscitation needs have been calculated as 12,000 mL/24 hours according to the burn/Baxter formula (4 mL of LR X kg body weight X TBSA burned), how many mL of fluid should be administered during the first 8 hours?

    a. 3000 mL.
    b. 4000 mL.
    c. 6000 mL.
    d. 9000 mL.

16. With massive hemorrhage and lack of adequate volumes of donor blood, which of the following patients is a candidate for autotransfusion?

    a. A patient with a large volume hemothorax associated with a malignant lesion.
    b. A patient with a large volume hemothorax from traumatic injury.
    c. A patient with a gunshot and shrapnel wounds to the abdomen with severe bleeding.
    d. Any patient with severe blood loss and no other available blood.

17. If a soccer player was hit in the head by the ball and showed signs of transient confusion for 10 minutes after the injury but then the confusion resolved, the concussion would be classified as

    a. Grade 1.
    b. Grade 2.
    c. Grade 3.
    d. Grade 4.

18. An adult patient has central venous pressure (CVP) monitoring, and the pressure is falling. Which procedure confirms suspected hypovolemia?

    a. Rapid fluid infusion of 250 to 500 mL and then evaluation in 10 minutes.
    b. Repeat readings every 5 minutes X 5 to determine further decrease in pressure.
    c. Decrease rate of IV fluids and observe for further decrease in pressure.
    d. Increase rate of fluids 2 X current rate and evaluate for increase in pressure.

19. The primary indications of mandibular fracture include

    a. dental avulsion and pain in mandibular area.
    b. malocclusion and ecchymosis of floor of the mouth.
    c. impaired sensation in chin and floor of mouth.
    d. pain and edema in chin and neck area.

20. A 30-year-old patient with an ipsilateral fracture of the distal radius and dislocation of the elbow complains of severe increasing pain in the forearm. The pain is unrelieved by analgesia. Which of the following should the nurse suspect?

    a. Infection.
    b. Fat embolism.
    c. Drug tolerance.
    d. Compartment syndrome.

21. A patient has had a long-leg plaster cast applied to the left leg after a skiing accident that resulted in a fractured tibia and fibula. The cast is still damp, but the patient complains that the cast feels hot and uncomfortable. Which of the following does the feeling of heat most likely indicate?

   a. Infection.
   b. Ill-fitting cast.
   c. Normal reaction.
   d. Anxiety.

22. Upon arrival at the trauma center, a pregnant woman is about to deliver but the umbilical cord is prolapsed. What position should the woman be placed in to relieve pressure on the cord?

   a. Supine.
   b. Knees to chest.
   c. Left lateral.
   d. Right lateral.

23. When assessing the ABCDEs of a patient with a traumatic brain injury, indications of Cushing's triad (bradycardia, hypertension, and abnormal irregular respirations) may be a sign of

   a. brainstem herniation.
   b. cerebral hemisphere damage.
   c. dilation of ventricles.
   d. decreased intracerebral pressure.

24. A patient with blunt trauma to the lower jaw and suspected mandibular fracture should first be assessed for

   a. airway obstruction.
   b. tooth loss.
   c. hemorrhage.
   d. sensory changes.

25. Which of the following is the purpose of defusing sessions in critical incident stress management (CISM)?

   a. Allow people to express feelings.
   b. Provide a critique of the stress-inducing event.
   c. Educate and provide guidance in handling feelings.
   d. Identify signs of stress.

26. One hour after an emergency delivery of a term infant, palpation of the mother's fundus shows that it is firm but deviates from midline. What should the trauma nurse suspect is the cause?

   a. Uterine bleeding.
   b. Bladder distention.
   c. Normal variation.
   d. Uterine rupture.

27. A patient suffered cardiac trauma with tamponade and has an emergent unguided pericardiocentesis with ECG monitoring. As the needle is advanced and blood withdrawn, premature ventricular contractions (PVCs) occur. What does this most likely indicate?

    a. Normal response to reduction in pressure.
    b. Acute injury to myocardium.
    c. Laceration of peritoneum.
    d. Irritation of the epicardium.

28. A patient with a basilar skull fracture is especially at risk of

    a. seizures.
    b. hemorrhage.
    c. cerebrospinal fluid leakage.
    d. airway obstruction.

29. In the ATLS protocol for trauma, during which step is a complete physical examination done, including neurological assessment and defining of disability?

    a. Primary survey.
    b. Resuscitation.
    c. Secondary survey.
    d. Definitive treatment.

30. The "death triangle" associated with rapid volume resuscitation and transfusions for treatment of hypovolemic shock includes acidosis (metabolic), coagulopathy, and which of the following?

    a. Cerebral edema.
    b. Hypothermia.
    c. Increased hemorrhage.
    d. Pulmonary edema.

31. A 14-year-old child with brain trauma presents with status epilepticus and a series of tonic-clonic seizures with intervening time too short for the child to regain consciousness. Which initial treatment is indicated?

    a. Rapid sequence intubation.
    b. Acyclovir and ceftriaxone.
    c. Phenytoin and phenobarbitol.
    d. Fast-acting benzodiazepine, such as Ativan®.

32. A patient who experienced facial trauma has epistaxis from tearing of posterior vessels of the nose. The most likely treatment is

    a. local pressure.
    b. nasal vasoconstrictive spray.
    c. compression tamponade.
    d. cold compresses.

33. A 30-year-old football player experienced a dislocation of the right knee and is in the emergency department with the knee splinted. Which of the following assessments has priority?

    a. Vascular assessment.
    b. Nerve function assessment.
    c. Pain evaluation.
    d. Assessment for further injuries to tendons, ligaments, and cartilage.

34. A 27-year-old patient is admitted to the emergency room with an open contaminated fracture of the tibia following a tractor accident. Which of the following information is especially important to obtain from the patient?

    a. Cause of accident.
    b. Date of last treatment with antibiotics.
    c. Description of environment where accident occurred.
    d. Date of last tetanus shot.

35. A 70-year-old patient with fracture of the proximal femur develops sudden onset of hypoxia, tachypnea, high fever, buccal and conjunctival petechiae, and tachycardia 24 hours after injury. Initial arterial blood gases indicate respiratory alkalosis. Which of the following possible complications is most likely the cause of these symptoms?

    a. Venous thromboembolia.
    b. Infection.
    c. Hemorrhage.
    d. Fat embolism syndrome (FES).

36. For a patient with contained blunt aortic injury but multiple other injuries that require delay in surgical repair, antihypertensives are administered to maintain systolic blood pressure below

    a. 80 mm Hg.
    b. 100 mm Hg.
    c. 120 mm Hg.
    d. 140 mm Hg.

37. Which of the following fractures poses the greatest risk of hypovolemic shock?

    a. Humerus.
    b. Tibia.
    c. Clavicle.
    d. Femur.

38. If an adult patient has second- and third-degree burns of both arms (front and back), the front of the trunk, and the perineum, using the rule of 9s, what percentage of total body surface area (TBSA) is burned?

    a. 37%.
    b. 45%.
    c. 46%.
    d. 55%.

39. A patient with a fractured vertebra is experiencing severe muscle spasms. Which of the following treatments is likely to offer the most relief?

    a. Cold to fractured area.

    b. Opioid analgesia.

    c. Position change.

    d. Heat to fractured area.

40. A patient has small shards of glass lodged in the surface of both corneas. After instillation of a topical anesthetic, the foreign bodies are usually removed with a

    a. small hemostat.

    b. pair of tweezers.

    c. 21-gauge needle.

    d. folded gauze pad.

41. The most common traumatic intracerebral lesion is the

    a. epidural hematoma.

    b. subdural hematoma.

    c. subarachnoid hemorrhage

    d. intracerebral hemorrhage.

42. A physician has ordered that a patient with an unstable pelvic fracture have a Foley catheter inserted into the bladder. Which of the following should be done prior to insertion of the Foley?

    a. Urinalysis.

    b. Cystoscopy.

    c. Intravenous pyelogram.

    d. Retrograde urethrogram.

43. A patient with compression fractures of the thoracic and lumbar region has been prescribed a thoracolumbosacral orthosis (TLSO) brace with metal sternal attachment. After logrolling the patient to sitting position, which should the trauma nurse assist the patient to do first?

    a. Put on a tight-fitting t-shirt.

    b. Place one arm through the straps on one side.

    c. Center the metal sternal attachment.

    d. Fasten the lumbar support.

44. A volleyball player slipped and fell hard, resulting in vertebral herniation at level L4—L5. For which of the following conditions is the patient most at risk?

    a. Cauda equina syndrome.

    b. Autonomic dysreflexia.

    c. Paraplegia.

    d. Spinal cord shock.

45. When determining the burden of proof for acts of negligence, how would risk management classify willfully providing inadequate care while disregarding the safety and security?

    a. Negligent conduct.

    b. Gross negligence.

    c. Contributory negligence.

    d. Comparative negligence.

46. A trauma victim has fractures of the upper 2 ribs on the right side. The patient should be carefully assessed for which secondary injury or injuries?

    a. Liver trauma.
    b. Splenic trauma.
    c. Tracheal/Bronchial/Great vessel trauma.
    d. Cardiac and splenic trauma.

47. Ensuring that a patient has given informed consent and understands his or her rights and all of the risks and benefits of a procedure or treatment supports the ethical principal of

    a. beneficence.
    b. nonmaleficence.
    c. justice.
    d. autonomy.

48. A trauma patient exhibits chest pain, pulsus paradoxus and Beck's triad: increased central venous pressure with distended neck veins, muffled heart sounds, and hypotension. Which of the following interventions is indicated?

    a. Angioplasty.
    b. Pericardiocentesis.
    c. Transmyocardial revascularization.
    d. Cardioversion.

49. A patient is suspected of having compartment syndrome associated with abdominal trauma and shock. Intraabdominal pressure is usually assessed by inserting

    a. a Foley catheter attached to a pressure transducer into the bladder.
    b. an NG tube attached to a pressure transducer into the stomach.
    c. a needle attached to a transducer into the abdominal fascia.
    d. an enteral tube attached to a transducer into the jejunum.

50. A patient who receives multiple transfusions with citrated blood products must be monitored closely for

    a. hyponatremia.
    b. hypomagnesemia.
    c. hypokalemia.
    d. hypocalcemia.

51. When irrigating a wound, what wound irrigation pressure is needed to effectively cleanse the wound while avoiding trauma?

    a. <4 psi.
    b. 20-30 psi.
    c. 10-15 psi.
    d. >15 psi.

52. A 25-year-old patient with multiple fractures from an auto accident develops hypoxia, dyspnea, precordial chest pain, tachycardia, and thick milky sputum. Auscultation of the lungs shows crackles and wheezes. The patient complains of headache and has a fever of 40°C. Which of the following interventions should be done first?

    a. High-flow oxygen.
    b. Corticosteroids (IV).
    c. Vasopressors.
    d. Morphine.

53. An 80-year-old patient has no insurance but is brought to the trauma center of a private hospital after a motor vehicle accident. The patient is hypovolemic and unstable, but the physician wants to transfer the patient. Which of the following acts should the trauma nurse cite as a reason to stop the transfer until the patient stabilizes?

    a. The Health Insurance Portability and Accountability Act (HIPAA).
    b. The Emergency Medical Treatment and Active Labor Act (EMTALA).
    c. American's with Disabilities Act (ADA).
    d. Older American Act (OAA).

54. A 3-year old girl has a spiral fracture of the shaft of her right humerus and numerous bruises, ranging from purple to yellow-green to brown, on her arms, legs, and face. The parent states that the child fell off of a swing set while playing the previous evening. The most appropriate action is

    a. contact Child Protective Services.
    b. caution the parent to supervise the child during play.
    c. ask the child what happened.
    d. tell the parent you suspect child abuse.

55. A 72-year-old female on Medicare is being discharged home with a healing burn on her left arm that she is unable to care for independently because of arthritis. She requires dressing changes every 3 days. She depends on public transportation and walks with difficulty. The bus stop is two blocks from her house. Her 12-year old granddaughter lives with her. The best solution is

    a. transferring the patient to an extended care facility.
    b. providing treatment on an outpatient basis at the hospital clinic.
    c. teaching the woman's 12-year-old granddaughter to do the dressing changes.
    d. making a referral to a home health agency to provide in-home care.

56. A blood specimen is obtained from a patient with a suspected highly infectious pathogen. Procedures should include which from the following?

    I. Notifying the lab in advance so they can take extra precautions.
    II. Labeling the vial as infectious.
    III. Placing the vial in a hazardous waste container for transport.
    IV. Discussing case with lab personnel prior to collection.

    a. I only
    b. I and II only
    c. I and IV only
    d. I, II, and III only

57. If a patient is on droplet precautions and no private room or cohorting is available, what minimum spatial separation should be maintained between the infected patient and a non-infected patient?

    a. six feet.
    b. four feet.
    c. three feet.
    d. two feet.

58. A patient with inhalation injury has a carboxyhemoglobin (COHB) level completed with initial lab work as part of evaluation for carbon monoxide (CO) poisoning. A normal percentage of COHB is

    a. <5%.
    b. <10%.
    c. <15%.
    d. <20%.

59. The most common type of transmission of infectious organisms in the healthcare facility is

    a. common source/vehicle.
    b. droplet
    c. airborne.
    d. contact.

60. If a patient receiving packed red blood cells develops febrile nonhemolytic reaction with chills, fever, headache, muscle ache, restlessness, and flushing, but BP and respiratory status remain stable, the reaction the patient is having is probably directed at the

    a. red blood cells.
    b. residual plasma.
    c. residual white blood cells.
    d. residual platelets.

61. Prehospital, a patient is found lying on the street with multiple stab wounds and the knife protruding from the right chest. During transport, the knife should be

    a. removed immediately.
    b. padded for support and left in place.
    c. removed if blood is oozing about the knife.
    d. held in place manually.

62. According to CDC guidelines, in the emergency response to a needlestick or a cut, the first action is to

    a. apply a disinfectant.
    b. notify a supervisor.
    c. irrigate the area with normal saline.
    d. wash the area with soap and water.

63. When looking at benchmarks, the trauma nurse notes that the trauma center ranks 69% in one category. This means that the center

    a. scored higher than 69% of those benchmarked against.
    b. scored lower than 69% of those benchmarked against.
    c. has an actual score of 31%.
    d. scored higher than 31% of those benchmarked against.

64. Plans to respond to acts of terrorism involving release of biologic agents should include

    I. developing a phone/email tree to notify all necessary staff and public health officials.
    II. stockpiling adequate personal protective equipment and respirators.
    III. developing procedures for handling of deaths.
    IV. establishing procedures for monitoring for air and water contamination.

    a. I and II only.
    b. I, III, and IV only.
    c. I, II, and IV only.
    d. I, II, III, and IV.

65. A gunshot wound to the intraperitoneal area of the abdomen increases risk of injury to

    a. pancreas and kidneys.
    b. ascending and descending colon.
    c. urinary bladder and rectum.
    d. liver and spleen.

66. When instructing families and visitors about methods to prevent and control infections, the best approach is to focus on their

    a. staying at least 3 feet away from patients.
    b. using proper hand hygiene before and after patient contact.
    c. reading literature about infection control.
    d. avoiding touching environmental surfaces.

67. When conducting a health history, the four most important areas to assess for a patient with musculoskeletal problems are

    a. pain, co-morbidities, swelling, and range of motion.
    b. age, goals, limitations, and pain.
    c. onset of symptoms, degree of pain, age, and range of motion.
    d. onset of symptoms, degree of deformity, paralysis/paresis, and pain.

68. A patient's $PaCO_2$ has shown an abrupt increase from 42 mm Hg to 52 mm Hg and the pH has decreased from 7.38 to 7.3 although the HCO_3 remains within normal limits. The most likely cause is

    a. acute respiratory acidosis.
    b. chronic respiratory acidosis.
    c. respiratory alkalosis.
    d. metabolic alkalosis.

69. A patient's external pulse oximeter is showing a decrease in SPO$_2$ to 80% although the patient does not appear to be in respiratory distress. The first step should be to

    a. request arterial blood gases.
    b. reposition the pulse oximeter.
    c. replace the pulse oximeter.
    d. place the pulse oximeter on the opposite side.

70. When teaching an older adult patient to use an MDI, the trauma nurse notes that the patient consistently fails to coordinate inhalation and actuation of the inhaler. The best solution for this patient is probably to

    a. ask the patient to practice for an extended period.
    b. print out directions for the patient.
    c. suggest the physician order a different type of inhaler or an adapter.
    d. repeat demonstration of use for the patient.

71. The "talk and die" phenomenon in which a patient loses consciousness after a blow to the head and then recovers and appears to be fine before suddenly developing severe symptoms of brain injury is typical of:

    a. epidural hemorrhage.
    b. subdural hemorrhage.
    c. intracerebral hemorrhage.
    d. subarachnoid hemorrhage.

72. Fifteen hours after a patient was involved in an automobile accident, the patient presents in the trauma center with abdominal discomfort and a positive Cullen's sign (bruising about the umbilicus). The trauma nurse should suspect

    a. ruptured spleen.
    b. retroperitoneal bleeding.
    c. hepatic laceration.
    d. ruptured diaphragm.

73. The most common cause of distributive shock is

    a. acute adrenal insufficiency.
    b. vasodilator drugs.
    c. anaphylaxis.
    d. sepsis.

74. Systemic inflammatory response syndrome (SIRS) is characterized by at least two indications, which may include

    a. changes in mental status and hypoxemia <72 mm Hg).
    b. bradycardia and tachypnea.
    c. elevated (>38° C) or subnormal (>36° C) rectal temperature.
    d. bradycardia and leukopenia (<4000).

75. A patient brought to the trauma center after a motorcycle accident exhibits bruising over the area of the mastoid process (Battle's sign) as well as otorrhea. These are indications of:

    a. cervical neck injury.
    b. basilar skull fracture.
    c. epidural hematoma.
    d. subarachnoid hemorrhage.

76. A patient with severe blunt trauma to the liver has received fluid resuscitation during transportation to the trauma center to treat hypotension and unstable condition. The patient is especially at risk of

    a. hemorrhage and hemodilution.
    b. sepsis.
    c. peripheral ischemia.
    d. compartment syndrome.

77. Which of the following types of fractures is likely to result in the greatest loss of blood?

    a. femur.
    b. pelvis.
    c. elbow.
    d. tibia.

78. Because there is only one bed available but two patients in need of care, the trauma nurse recommends that one patient be transferred to another facility. The decision regarding which patient to transfer should be based on which ethical principle?

    a. Nonmaleficence
    b. Beneficence.
    c. Justice.
    d. Autonomy.

79. A trauma patient has lost 15% to 25% (750-1500 mL) of total blood volume and exhibits tachycardia (110 bpm), prolonged capillary refill and increased diastolic BP. Respirations are 24 and urinary output is 25 mL/hr. This hemorrhagic shock is classified a:

    a. Class I.
    b. Class II.
    c. Class III.
    d. Class IV.

80. A patient presents in the emergency department after falling from a horse and being kicked in the left side. In addition to a fractured left lower rib, the patient exhibits elevation of the left hemidiaphragm, left lower lobe atelectasis, and pleural effusion as well as tachycardia, hypotension, left flank pain, and positive Kehr sign (pain referred to left shoulder). The trauma nurse recognizes these signs and symptoms as indications of

    a. ruptured spleen.
    b. hepatic trauma.
    c. gastric perforation.
    d. pancreatic trauma.

81. A patient who was the victim of a violent assault and rape is shaking and crying and appears terrified. Which of the following responses is most therapeutic at the initial encounter with the patient?

a. "Why are you crying?"
b. "I can see you are still frightened."
c. "What can I do to help you?"
d. "You are safe now."

82. What level (ACS designation) is a trauma center that has trauma nurse(s) and physician(s) available on patient arrival and can provide advanced life support and stabilization for transfer?

a. Level II.
b. Level III.
c. Level IV.
d. Level V.

83. A patient is airlifted to the hospital with a spinal cord injury and is not breathing independently. Total loss of respiratory muscle function occurs with spinal cord injuries above

a. C4.
b. C5.
c. C6.
d. C7

84. Which of the following procedures is most correct for the removal of clothing during an examination of a patient who has been assaulted?

a. All of the clothing should be placed in one large paper bag.
b. Each piece of clothing should be placed in a separate paper bag.
c. Clothing with stains or tears should be placed in one large paper bag.
d. Clothing with any potential evidence should be placed in one large paper bag.

85. When preparing to administer a unit of packed red blood cells, the trauma nurse notes gas bubbles in the blood. This may indicate

a. normal finding.
b. hemolysis.
c. excess plasma.
d. bacterial infection.

86. A 36-year-old female was injured in a fall when drunk. CT shows contusion on the left side of the brain. The patient responds lethargically to verbal commands and shows some confusion and restlessness. Vital signs: BP 154/76, pulse 68, and respirations 28. Previous records indicate her normal baseline BP was 128/70, pulse 76, and respirations 16. The change in VS is most likely an indication of

a. increasing intracranial pressure.
b. stress response.
c. ethanol intoxication.
d. delirium tremens.

87. A tornado has caused significant damage in a rural town and multiple injuries. The closest hospital is 150 miles away. Only one helicopter is available for transport, but ambulances are scheduled to arrive within 15 minutes. After triage, which of the following patients should be airlifted?

    a. 50-year old woman with first and second degree burns on arms and hands (12% of BSA).
    b. 12-year old boy with a fractured elbow.
    c. 25-year old woman at 24 weeks gestation in active labor.
    d. 45-year old man with penetrating trauma in his left leg from shards of wood.

88. When offloading a patient from a helicopter, receiving medical personnel should be advised to

    a. immediately approach the helicopter from the front.
    b. wait until the helicopter shuts down (about 2 minutes).
    c. approach the helicopter in a crouched position.
    d. approach the helicopter only when signaled to do so by crew.

89. The pediatric BIG (bone injection gun) for intraosseous infusion is intended for use only in the

    a. proximal tibia.
    b. proximal tibia or proximal humerus.
    c. proximal humerus.
    d. sternum.

90. At the site of an explosion, a patient with multiple shrapnel wounds in the left arm has severe uncontrolled bleeding. When placing a tourniquet to control bleeding during transit, the trauma nurse should

    a. examine the position of all wounds before placing the tourniquet immediately above.
    b. place the tourniquet 2 to 3 inches above area of most severe bleeding.
    c. place the tourniquet proximally ("high and tight") on the left arm.
    d. place the tourniquet about 6 inches above bleeding.

91. When attempting to control hemorrhage with permissive hypotension, in order to maintain adequate perfusion, the systolic blood pressure should not fall below

    a. 70 mm Hg.
    b. 80 mm Hg.
    c. 90 mm Hg.
    d. 100 mm Hg.

92. Which of the following is an indication for an open thoracotomy at bedside for a patient?

    a. Systolic BP <80 mm Hg despite resuscitation attempts.
    b. Non-traumatic cardiac arrest.
    c. Loss of 1600 mL blood per chest tube.
    d. Lack of witnessed cardiac activity.

93. In evaluating research as part of the development of evidence-based practice guidelines, the four evaluative/trustworthiness criteria are (1) credibility, (2) dependability, (3) transferability, and (4)

    a. controllability.
    b. applicability.
    c. accountability.
    d. confirmability.

94. A primary consideration of mortality and morbidity reviews is

a. assigning blame for errors.
b. determining punishment for negligent care.
c. improvement in the provision of care.
d. identifying cases involving substandard care.

95. If a patient involved in a motorcycle accident is maintained on life support but meets the criteria for brain death and does not carry an organ donor card, the trauma nurse's responsibility is generally to

a. ask the family for consent for donation.
b. ensure the organ procurement organization is notified.
c. discuss organ donation options with the family.
d. assume the patient would not want organ donation.

96. A visitor stops the trauma nurse and asks, "Could you tell me what happened to the patient across from my husband? He seems so agitated." The response that complies with the Health Insurance Portability and Accountability Act (HIPAA) is

a. "His wife is in the waiting area. You can go ask her."
b. "May I ask why are you asking?"
c. "The law doesn't allow me to give out any information about patients in order to protect their privacy and safety."
d. "He was involved in a motor vehicle accident, like your husband."

97. If a pregnant patient was involved in an automobile accident with abdominal trauma and experienced placental abruption, the patient must be carefully monitored for indications of

a. disseminated intravascular coagulopathy (DIC).
b. uterine rupture.
c. diaphragmatic rupture.
d. infection.

98. A patient that suffered severe blunt chest trauma resulting in fractured lower ribs is exhibiting hemidiaphragmatic elevation and atelectasis of the lower lobe of the left lung, suggesting

a. flail chest.
b. diaphragmatic injury.
c. pericardial effusion.
d. pulmonary contusion.

99. The trauma nurse is part of a committee evaluating the trauma center and assessing the need for change. Which of the following should be the primary focus when instituting change?

a. Current trends in medical care.
b. Staff preference.
c. Best available evidence-based research.
d. Community needs.

100. A patient is brought to the trauma center after an automobile accident. The patient has multiple fractured ribs and exhibits labored breathing with respiratory rate of 40/min. The patient's oxygen saturation is 86% and the patient is hemodynamically unstable. The trauma nurse should prepare the patient for

    a.   continuous positive airway pressure (CPAP).
    b.   intubation and mechanical ventilation.
    c.   hyperbaric oxygen therapy.
    d.   cardiopulmonary resuscitation.

101. A patient who accidentally amputated his hand in a chainsaw accident is brought to the trauma center by a friend with the amputated hand wrapped in a dry towel. After irrigating the hand with NS, the hand should be stored by being

    a.   wrapped with saline moistened dressing inside a sealed plastic bag and immersed in ice water.
    b.   wrapped with dry dressing inside a sealed plastic bag and immersed in ice water.
    c.   immersed directly into a container of ice water.
    d.   immersed directly into room temperature NS.

102. If a patient experienced a high voltage electrical shock with electrical burns from touching a live wire with the palm of his hand while standing and bending over, the trauma nurse would expect exit wounds

    a.   on the top of the hand.
    b.   on the feet.
    c.   at multiple sites.
    d.   at the proximal arm.

103. If extended focused abdominal sonography for trauma (eFAST) is being used to identify pneumothorax or hemothorax associated with blunt trauma, the probe should be placed at the

    a.   fourth intercostal space at the parasternal line.
    b.   second intercostal space at the parasternal line.
    c.   fourth intercostal space at the mid-clavicular line.
    d.   second intercostal space at the mid-clavicular line.

104. When placing an arterial line for a patient with hemodynamic instability, the preferred access site is the

    a.   femoral artery.
    b.   radial artery.
    c.   brachial artery.
    d.   dorsalis pedis artery.

105. When applying a pelvic stabilization device for a patient with a fractured pelvis, the circumferential pressure should be applied to the

    a.   suprapubic area.
    b.   mid-pubic area.
    c.   greater trochanter region.
    d.   iliac crests.

106. If using the ask-tell-ask framework to educate a patient and family about self-care, the trauma nurse would begin by

    a. waiting for the patient to ask a question.
    b. providing information and asking the patient to repeat it back.
    c. asking the patient to write down a number of questions.
    d. asking the patient what he/she knows and wants to know.

107. The 5 key elements of pain assessment include (1) words, (2) intensity, (3) location, (4) duration, and (5)

    a. method/administration
    b. aggravating/alleviating factors.
    c. frequency.
    d. quality.

108. A family reports that a trauma patient who was raised Catholic has not attended Mass for 50 years. The patient is nearing death but remains responsive and has not requested a priest. The trauma nurse should

    a. assume the patient will not want to see a priest.
    b. ask the priest on call to visit the patient.
    c. ask the patient if he or she wants to see a priest.
    d. ask the family if a priest should be called.

109. A 26-year-old male with no advance directive suffered a traumatic brain injury that left him in a vegetative state on life support. The patient's mother, sister, best friend, and fiancée are present. Which family member or other person can legally make the decision to withdraw life support?

    a. Friend.
    b. Sister.
    c. Mother.
    d. Fiancée.

110. A patient with blunt trauma to the genitals resulting from a physical assault has a fractured penis with gross hematuria. The trauma nurse should prepare the patient for which type of imaging?

    a. CT.
    b. FAST.
    c. MRI.
    d. RUG.

111. A patient with a blunt trauma neck injury has apparent laryngeal damage with subcutaneous emphysema and irregular contour of thyroid cartilage. The patient is sitting in tripod position to ease respiratory distress. The trauma nurse should anticipate that the airway will be secured by

    a. rapid-sequence intubation (oral).
    b. emergent surgical airway.
    c. CPAP with nasal administration.
    d. nasopharyngeal airway.

112. A trauma victim has fractures of the lower ribs (8 and 9) on the right side. The patient should be carefully assessed for which secondary injury or injuries?

   a. Liver trauma.
   b. Splenic trauma.
   c. Tracheal/Bronchial/Great vessel trauma.
   d. Cardiac and splenic trauma.

113. Based on research of best practices, the trauma nurse has recommended a number of best practice guidelines to improve patient safety and patient outcomes. Which type of best practice should the trauma nurse generally attempt to institute first?

   a. A practice that requires new equipment.
   b. A practice that involves the entire staff.
   c. A practice that requires organizational change.
   d. A practice that requires simple changes in procedure.

114. A patient with a traumatic chest injury and multiple fractured ribs has shown increasing evidence of mild to moderate pulmonary contusion with slowly increasing hypoxemia and hemoptysis. The goal of fluid resuscitation in the presence of pulmonary contusion is

   a. hypovolemia.
   b. euvolemia.
   c. hypervolemia.
   d. unrelated to pulmonary contusion.

115. When checking compartment pressure in the volar compartment of the forearm using the Stryker Intracompartmental pressure monitor device, the pressure reading that indicates onset of compartment syndrome is

   a. >15 mm Hg.
   b. >20 mm Hg.
   c. >30 mm Hg.
   d. >40 mm Hg.

116. Massive transfusion protocol (MTP) is usually activated if a patient's anticipated use of PRBCs is

   a. ≥3 units in <4 hours.
   b. ≥4 units in <4 hours.
   c. ≥6 units in <4 hours.
   d. ≥8 units in <4 hours.

117. Which of the following would be excluded from a trauma registry?

   a. Severe myocardial infarction.
   b. Gunshot wound.
   c. Motor vehicle injury.
   d. Stabbing injury.

118. Which of the following governmental agencies provides safety standards for the workplace and workers?

   a. FEMA.
   b. FDA.
   c. OSHA.
   d. FLSA.

119. If a patient has ingested sodium hydroxide, the immediate response after ensuring airway patency should be to

   a. induce vomiting.
   b. administer activated charcoal.
   c. administer antacid.
   d. administer one-half to one cup of milk or water.

120. A patient with spinal cord injury at T4 has developed bradycardia, hypotension, and autonomic instability. These indications suggest the patient is developing

   a. autonomic dysreflexia.
   b. neurogenic shock.
   c. sepsis.
   d. distributive shock.

121. A patient with septic shock has progressed to multi-organ dysfunction syndrome (MODS) and has developed thrombocytopenia, increasing the patient's risk of

   a. disseminated intravascular coagulation.
   b. acute respiratory distress syndrome.
   c. renal failure.
   d. bowel necrosis.

122. If a patient with a soft tissue infection of the foot that occurred following an accidental cut has developed severe pain, erythema, tense edema, and crepitus as well as hypotension, tachycardia, and elevated temperature, the most critical emergent treatment is

   a. antibiotic therapy.
   b. IV fluid resuscitation.
   c. negative pressure therapy.
   d. surgical debridement.

123. An Rh- patient who is 7 months pregnant is involved in an automobile accident and experienced blunt abdominal trauma from the abdomen hitting the steering wheel. The fetus does not appear to be in distress and the mother's injuries are minor although the mother has experienced some mild irregular contractions. The patient should be

   a. discharged and advised to see an obstetrician for follow up.
   b. administered a tocolytic.
   c. administered Rh-immune globulin.
   d. administered magnesium sulfate.

124. A patient with a fractured pelvis from blunt trauma has gross hematuria and CT cystography shows an extraperitoneal rupture of the bladder. The most likely initial treatment for the bladder injury is

a. wait and watch.
b. insertion of Foley catheter with continuous drainage.
c. surgical repair.
d. antibiotics.

125. The primary purpose of using the SBAR (situation, background, assessment, recommendations) format for hands-off when transferring a patient from the trauma center to a different department is to

a. improve patient safety.
b. meet regulatory requirements.
c. simplify transitions.
d. save time.

126. The trauma center has experienced a number of patient falls resulting in injuries. The first step in preventing falls is to

a. routinely ensure side rails are up and beds low.
b. maintain patient visibility.
c. ensure call light is easily accessible.
d. carry out routine risk assessments.

127. Which of the following interventions is most likely to reduce nursing injuries?

a. Zero-lift policy.
b. Increased security personnel.
c. Mandatory reporting of injuries.
d. Eight-hour shifts instead of 12-hour.

128. When beginning the chain of collection with recovery of a bullet from a gunshot wound, the three elements that must be included in addition to patient name/identifying number and signature of collecting practitioner are (1) description of item, (2) date and time of recovery, and (3)

a. size of item recovered.
b. location where it was recovered.
c. names of all witnesses to recovery.
d. manner of collection.

129. If a train crash occurs with multiple injuries and deaths and the triage team is using the black-red-yellow-green triage classification system for tagging victims, the trauma nurse would ensure the first patients to receive care are those tagged with

a. black.
b. green.
c. yellow.
d. red.

130. If a 5-year-old child cries frantically when the parents are present but quiets when the parents leave the bedside, the trauma nurse should

a. encourage the parents to stay in the waiting area.
b. reassure the parents that this is normal healthy response.
c. assume the child is crying due to fear of potentially abusive parents.
d. assume the child is trying to get attention.

131. If a 16-year-old female patient is seriously injured but alert and responsive and the trauma nurse needs to find out if the patient may be pregnant but the parents are with the patient, the trauma nurse should

a. ask the patient in the presence of the parents.
b. ask the parents if the patient might be pregnant.
c. ask the parents to step outside briefly and ask the patient in privacy.
d. examine the patient for indications of pregnancy.

132. Which of the following symbols indicate a possible health hazard and could include carcinogens, toxic substances, and respiratory irritants?

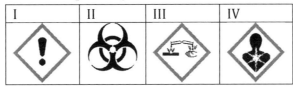

a. I.
b. II.
c. III.
d. IV.

133. For patients with penetrating abdominal trauma, the three aspect of damage control/hemostatic resuscitation include (1) early activating of massive transfusion protocol, (2) avoiding the use of large volume crystalloid administration, and (3) utilizing

a. early laparotomy.
b. permissive hypotension.
c. FAST.
d. antibiotic prophylaxis.

134. A patient has second-degree burns on both hands with blistering and sloughing of outer layers of skin. Which initial pain control method is generally preferred?

a. IV morphine.
b. Transdermal fentanyl patch.
c. Oral hydrocodone.
d. Soaking hands in ice water.

135. When using waveform capnography (end-tidal CO_2) to assess ventilation in a patient with a head injury, a normal finding is

a. 15 to 25 mm Hg.
b. 25 to 35 m Hg.
c. 35 to 45 mm Hg.
d. 45 to 55 mm Hg.

136. A patient who sustained a blunt thoracic injury when hit in the chest by a hardball while playing baseball is admitted with severe chest pain, but the patient suddenly develops the below rhythm. What does this ECG rhythm strip indicate?

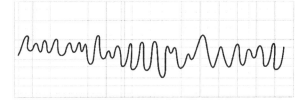

- a. Supraventricular tachycardia.
- b. Atrial flutter.
- c. Ventricular tachycardia.
- d. Ventricular fibrillation.

137. If a patient experiences a distal fracture of the radius, the patient is at risk for neurovascular injury of the

- a. radial nerve.
- b. median nerve.
- c. ulnar nerve.
- d. axillary nerve.

138. With a stab wound to the abdomen, the organ that is most frequently injured is the

- a. liver.
- b. colon.
- c. small intestine.
- d. diaphragm.

139. The most effective laboratory tests when assessing oxygenation and onset of shock in a patient who is bleeding heavily are

- a. hemoglobin and hematocrit.
- b. hematocrit and platelet count.
- c. blood gases.
- d. coagulation studies.

140. In an unstable patient with blunt abdominal trauma, the preferred method of screening is

- a. plain radiography.
- b. DPL.
- c. CT scan.
- d. FAST.

141. If a patient receiving blood transfusions shows signs of a mild allergic reaction, including pruritis, erythema, and urticaria, the usual treatment is to stop the transfusion and administer

- a. antihistamine.
- b. epinephrine.
- c. corticosteroids.
- d. vasopressin.

142. Which of the following is the preferred site for placement of a central line?

    a. Left internal jugular vein.
    b. Right internal jugular vein.
    c. Femoral vein.
    d. Subclavian vain.

143. A Salem sump tube is inserted nasogastrically for a patient with bowel obstruction in order to decompress the stomach, which is painful and distended. Following insertion, the trauma nurse aspirates gastric fluids to check pH values. Which of the following values is consistent with gastric fluids?

    a. 7.2.
    b. 5.7.
    c. 4.5.
    d. 3.8.

144. If a patient is involved in an accident with injury to the occipital lobe (coup injury), the other part of the brain that likely experienced injury (contrecoup) is the

    a. frontal lobe.
    b. midbrain.
    c. parietal area.
    d. temporal area.

145. If a patient was involved in a football injury with a concussion resulting from impact to the temporal lobe, typical indications include

    a. bizarre behavior.
    b. visual disturbance.
    c. disorientation/amnesia.
    d. gait disturbances.

146. If a patient with a pneumothorax is hemodynamically stable and the physician is preparing to carry out needle decompression in the midclavicular line, the trauma nurse should prep the skin at the

    a. fifth and/or sixth intercostal space.
    b. third and/or fourth intercostal space.
    c. second and/or third intercostal space.
    b. first and/or second intercostal space.

147. The three elements involved in establishing the mechanism of injury include

    a. questioning/listening, observation, and physical examination.
    b. looking, touching, and listening.
    c. physical examination, laboratory/imaging, and type of injury.
    d. laboratory, Imaging, and physical examination.

148. When providing discharge education to an adolescent who experienced a second grade 2 concussion, the adolescent should be advised that participating in sports should be avoided until after follow up with neurosurgeon and for at least

    a. one week after asymptomatic.
    b. two weeks after asymptomatic.
    c. one month after asymptomatic.
    d. two months after asymptomatic.

149. A patient who identified as a Jehovah Witness needs a transfusion of packed red blood cells because of blood loss, but his religion prohibits blood transfusions. Which of the following is the correct action?

    a. Assume the patient will not accept a transfusion and report this to the physician.
    b. Tell the patient that he may die without the transfusion.
    c. Tell the patient that his health is more important than religious beliefs.
    d. Provide full information and the reasons for the transfusion.

150. Which of the following is a legal document that specifically designates someone to make decisions regarding medical and end-of-life care if a patient is mentally incompetent?

    a. Advance directive.
    b. Do-not-resuscitate order.
    c. Durable Power of Attorney.
    d. General Power of Attorney.

151. Adult patients with abdominal trauma that necessitates a splenectomy should receive which vaccination?

    a. Hepatitis B.
    b. Tetanus.
    c. Human papillomavirus.
    d. Polyvalent pneumococcal.

152. If a patient has suffered from hypothermia with reduced core temperature to 30° C, rewarming should be done at the rate of

    a. 0.5 to 1° C per 0.5 hr.
    b. 0.5 to 1° C per hr.
    c. 1 to 2° C per hr.
    d. 3 to 4° C per hr.

153. If a patient experienced a blunt impact sports-related scrotal injury and presents with severe pain and swelling of the scrotum, for what type of imaging should the trauma nurse prepare the patient?

    a. Ultrasound.
    b. Radiograph.
    c. CT.
    d. MRI.

154. A severely mangled extremity is likely to require amputation if the score on the Mangled Extremity Severity Scoring (MESS) is greater than

a. 12.
b. 9.
c. 7.
d. 5.

155. A normal prothrombin time is

a. 21 to 35 seconds.
b. 10 to 15 seconds.
c. 30 to 45 seconds.
d. 2 to 9.5 minutes.

156. When teaching a patient incision care prior to discharge, the best technique to ensure the patient understands is

a. ask the patient to give a return demonstration.
b. give the patient a brief quiz.
c. ask the patient to explain the procedure.
d. provide written directions for the patient to refer to.

157. When assessing skeletal or soft tissue injury, a stab wound would be classified as

a. very high energy.
b. high energy.
c. medium energy.
d. low energy.

158. When carrying out the apnea test on a patient to determine brain death, once the patient is off of the ventilator, the test should be aborted when the oxygen saturation falls to

a. <95%.
b. <93%.
c. <90%.
d. <85%.

159. Intracranial pressure monitoring is usually indicated for patients with traumatic brain injury and Glasgow Coma Score of

a. ≤4
b. ≤6
c. ≥8.
d. ≤10.

160. A 25-year-old patient with severe neurological injury and brain death is being maintained on life support until the organs can be recovered for donation. Which of the following tests is indicated prior to organ recovery?

a. coronary angiograms.
b. echocardiogram.
c. coronary calcium CT.
d. chest radiograph.

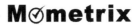

161. If a nursing diagnosis for a patient with a crush injury to the right leg is "risk for ineffective tissue perfusion," an expected patient outcome to interventions is

    a. distal limb dusky.
    b. tissue cool to touch.
    c. Color pale.
    d. capillary refill time 3 seconds.

162. An open irregular wound resulting from the tissue tearing in response to blunt trauma is classified as a(n)

    a. laceration.
    b. incision.
    c. avulsion.
    d. penetration.

163. If a physician has ordered negative pressure wound therapy (NPWT) for a patient, which of the following is a contraindication to the treatment?

    a. Copious purulent drainage.
    b. Exposed vessels.
    c. Arterial ulcers.
    d. Diabetic ulcers.

164. Which of the following patients is most likely to receive fluid resuscitation with isotonic IV fluids?

    a. A patient with pulmonary edema.
    b. A patient with increasing intracranial pressure.
    c. A patient with extracellular fluid loss associated with bleeding.
    d. A patient in diabetic ketoacidosis.

165. A trauma patient needs emergent surgery but has been receiving warfarin for atrial fibrillation. Prior to surgery, how is reversal of anticoagulation achieved?

    a. Administration of vitamin K and fresh frozen plasma.
    b. Administration of platelets.
    c. Administration of vitamin K.
    d. Reversal is not necessary.

166. A 76-year-old patient has a severe head injury. The caregiver reports that the patient fell. Physical examination shows multiple bruises in various stages of healing and a review of the patient's history shows 5 visits to the emergency department over the previous 18 months for minor to moderate injuries (cuts, fractures, bruising). The patient's appearance is unkempt, and the patient is very thin. The trauma nurse should suspect

    a. a bleeding disorder.
    b. cognitive impairment.
    c. elder abuse.
    d. negligence.

167. If a patient involved in a motor vehicle accident has typical lap-belt contusions (lap belt sign) and fracture of a lumbar vertebrae, the internal structure that is primarily at risk of contusion or transection is the

    a. aorta.
    b. pancreas.
    c. liver.
    d. spleen.

168. A 35-year old female involved in a side-impact automobile collision suffered pronounced cervical rotation and complains of severe right-sided neck pain and severe unremitting right-sided headache and exhibits ecchymosis and swelling of the right neck and right ophthalmic ptosis with contraction of the pupil (miosis). Which is the most likely reason for the symptoms?

    a. Herniated cervical disc.
    b. Carotid dissection.
    c. Neck strain.
    d. Spinal cord injury.

169. A patient is to have an intracranial monitoring device inserted that allows for CSF drainage and sampling. Which of the following devices is appropriate?

    a. Subarachnoid bolt/screw.
    b. Fiberoptic transducer-tipped catheter.
    c. Subdural/epidural catheter.
    d. Intraventricular catheter.

170. A patient who fell off of a 12-foot ladder onto a concrete floor complains of chest pain and pain in the posterior scapula area. The trauma nurse notes asymmetry in blood pressure of upper extremities, and upper extremity hypertension with a widened pulse pressure. Chest x-ray shows fracture of the scapulae and widened mediastinum (10 cm). Based on these findings, the trauma nurse suspects

    a. rupture of the aorta.
    b. cardiac tamponade.
    c. diaphragmatic injury.
    d. tracheobronchial injury.

171. If a pregnant patient dies from traumatic injuries at 34 weeks of gestation and the mother is provided continuous CPR, perimortem Cesarean to save the fetus must be carried out within

    a. 5 minutes.
    b. 15 minutes.
    c. 30 minutes.
    d. 60 minutes.

172. A 76-year-old female patient who has generally been in good health has suffered a pathological fracture of the proximal femur. The patient states it occurred while walking, resulting in a fall. The most likely cause is

    a. abuse.
    b. multiple myeloma.
    c. osteoporosis.
    d. bone cyst.

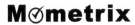

173. If a dying patient tells the trauma nurse that she sees her mother, who has been deceased for many years, the most appropriate response is

    a. "Does seeing your mother comfort or frighten you?"
    b. "You are just dreaming."
    c. "I'm sure your mother is watching over you."
    d. "It's probably because of the medicine."

174. If a patient has spinal cord injury resulting from a gunshot wound, reflex testing for L4 injury is carried out at the

    a. biceps.
    b. triceps.
    c. ankle.
    d. knee.

175. Which of the following procedures is used to evaluate the function of cranial nerve XI (spinal accessory) for a patient with a traumatic neck injury?

    a. Ask the patient to raise both eyebrows and frown.
    b. Place hands on patient's shoulders and ask the patient to shrug against resistance.
    c. Touch the patient's cornea with a fine piece of cotton and observe for blink response.
    d. Ask patient to swallow, speak, and say "Ahhh."

Answer Key and Explanations

1. B: When monitoring intracranial pressure in an adult, the trauma nurse must be aware that the normal range is 10 to 15 mm Hg. If bleeding occurs within the brain, the brain first attempts to compensate by decreasing the volume of CSF through increased absorption and decreasing blood flow, but when the brain can no longer compensate, the ICP begins to rise very rapidly, resulting in compression of the tissue and sometimes brain shift and herniation syndromes. If the condition is not immediately reversed, it can result in death within a very short period of time.

2. D: With a gunshot wound to the abdomen, the trauma nurse should anticipate that the organ most likely to be injured is the small intestine (half of injuries). However, depending on the trajectory and penetrance of the bullet, multiple other organs (such as the colon, liver, and major vessels) may also be injured. High energy gunshot wounds from close range may result in both primary injuries and secondary injuries, such as from bone fragments.

3. A: Mannitol administration for treatment of cerebral edema may result in fluid and electrolyte imbalance with hyperkalemia, which can cause cardiac arrhythmias. Mannitol is an osmotic diuretic that increases excretion of both sodium and water, increasing potassium levels, and reduces intracranial pressure and brain mass, especially after traumatic brain injury. Other side effects include nausea, vomiting, hypotension, tachycardia, fever, and urticaria. Mannitol may also be used to shrink the cells of the blood-brain barrier in order to help other medications breach this barrier. Cerebral spinal fluid pressure should show decrease within 15 minutes of administration.

4. C: If a handgun is found in the pocket of a trauma victim, the first consideration when removing and securing the gun is to avoid touching the trigger. All guns should be considered loaded even if assured it is empty of bullets. The gun should be removed wearing gloves and handled carefully to avoid disrupting fingerprints or gun powder residue and should be placed in a secure container, never a paper bag. When moving the gun, the barrel should never be pointed at others. If the gun has a safety device, it should be engaged.

5. B: If a patient with facial fractures has dentoalveolar trauma with avulsion of permanent teeth, reimplantation should ideally be carried out within 30 minutes because saving the tooth is often not possible after two hours or if the root is desiccated. If teeth cannot be immediately reimplanted, then they should be stored in a moist environment, such as in NS. Pediatric deciduous teeth are generally not reimplanted because of high failure rate and possible damage to underlying permanent teeth.

6. A: When utilizing the AMPLE acronym to rapidly obtain important information about the patient's history, the letter L stands for "Last meal." The information obtained is that which is essential to providing emergent care to the patient. If the patient is unable to respond, a family member or friend may provide information:

> A = Allergies.
> M = Medications (all current).
> P = Prior illnesses and surgeries.
> L = Last meal (time, size, contents).
> E = Events/Environment associated with the injury.

7. D: Acute subdural hematoma, which is most common in children <1 and often results from falls, impact, or abuse, is an emergent situation requiring immediate surgical evacuation of the hematoma as it presses directly on the brain and can lead to death. An ICP device may be inserted during surgery to monitor

155

pressure. Mannitol is an osmotic diuretic that increases excretion of sodium and water and reduces ICP related to traumatic brain injury. Hypertonic saline solution reduces hyponatremia, cerebral edema, and increased intracranial pressure associated with traumatic brain injury.

8. C: The non-rebreather mask, which covers the mouth and nose with a reservoir bag of oxygen, has a one-way valve that prevents the patient from rebreathing exhaled air and delivers FIO_2 of 60% to 80% or even higher at flow rates of 15 LPM. Partial rebreather masks provide 30% to 40% FIO_2 with oxygen flow between 6 and 12 LPM. Venturi masks provide 24% to 50% FIO_2 but FIO_2 is often unreliable over 35%. Nasal cannulas provide 24% to 40% FIO_2 and ≤6 LPM.

9. A: Most patients with a Glasgow coma score of 13 to 15 and mild to moderate head injuries do not require ICP monitoring. Those with severe head injury (even with a normal CT) usually require monitoring if they are >40, exhibit posturing, and are hypotensive (<90 systolic). ICP monitoring may be indicated with subarachnoid and intraventricular hemorrhage, cerebrovascular accident, brain tumors, brain abscesses/infections, and hydrocephalus. ICP threshold value for adults is 20 to 25 mm HG and for children, 20 mm Hg.

10. D: Apnea is an absolute contraindication to nasotracheal intubation. The primary indications are suspected or confirmed cervical spine injury resulting in a clenched jaw but with the gag reflex intact and severe respiratory distress. Facial and skull fractures may, in some cases, be contraindications, depending on the location and extent of fractures. The nares size must be adequate to accept endotracheal tube in sizes 7 to 8. Usually an anti-decongestant, such as phenylephrine 0.5 mg, is administered to the nostril prior to tube insertion.

11. D: With targeted temperature management (TTM), AKA therapeutic hypothermia, the patient's temperature should generally be lowered and maintained at 32 to 36° C. (Normal temperature is about 37° C). TTM is typically maintained for about 24 hours. Hypothermia is contraindicated in the presence of sepsis, recent surgery (within 2 weeks), coagulopathy, or pre-existing coma. Cooling may be achieved with ice packs, cooling blankets and/or helmets, and cool infusions or instillations.

12. B: Horizontal/lateral violence occurs when a colleague or peer uses intimidation, verbal abuse, rudeness, or even physical attacks toward another. People may blame others or bully them into complying with their demands. Horizontal violence may be overt or covert. Horizontal violence serves to erode self-confidence and makes a hostile work environment, increasing absenteeism and lowering staff morale. Studies show that more than half of nurses have experienced horizontal violence in the workplace. Each institution should have a code of conduct and a plan in place for dealing with horizontal violence.

13. D: If the paramedic reports that a patient in transit has a Glasgow Coma Score of 7, the trauma nurse expects the patient to be intubated and comatose. Scores of 8 or less indicate severe brain injury and have high risk of death. Intracranial pressure is often elevated. GSCs range from 3 (lowest and most severe) to 15 (best score):

- Mild: 13-15. Brief loss of consciousness.
- Moderate: 9-12. Confused but able to follow simple directions, possible focal neurological deficits.
- Severe ≤8. Comatose and requires ventilatory support, survivor likely have neurological impairment.

14. A: Rapid sequence intubation (RSI) is used to anesthetize and intubate the non-fasting patient to reduce risk of gastric aspiration. RSI may also be used for pregnant patients, very obese patients, and those with gastric reflux. Two intravenous lines should be in place prior to RSI and the patient preoxygenated for ≥3 minutes. Sellick's maneuver (pressure applied externally with thumb and index finger to cricoid) is used to close off the esophagus and prevent aspiration. An induction agent (thiopental, Entamide®, propofol) is followed by a muscle relaxant (suxamethonium). Sixty seconds after the muscle relaxant, an endotracheal tube is inserted with a laryngoscopy, cuff inflated and secured and placement verified by capnometer.

15. C: If a burn patient's fluid resuscitation needs have been calculated as 12,000 mL/24 hours according to the burn/Baxter formula (4 mL of LR X kg body weight X TBSA burned), 6000 mL of fluid (50% of total) should be administered during the first 8 hours and the remaining 6000 mL over the next 16 hours. Fluid resuscitation is indicated with burns of 20% or more of total body surface area (TBSA) burned. Lactated Ringers IV solution is used instead of NS, which can lead to hypernatremia and hyperchloremia.

16. B: With massive hemorrhage and lack of adequate volume of donor blood, a patient with a large volume hemothorax from traumatic injury is a candidate for autotransfusion. Blood is collected from a body cavity, most often the pleural cavity. Autotransfusion is contraindicated if malignant lesions are present in area of blood loss, pooled blood is contaminated (such as with fecal material), or wounds are >4-6 hours old. Commercial collection/transfusion kits (Pleur-Evac®, Thora-Klex®) are available but blood can be collected through the chest tube into a sterile bottle.

17. A: If a soccer player was hit in the head by the ball and showed signs of transient confusion for 10 minutes after the injury but then the confusion resolved, the concussion would be classified as Grade 1. There are 3 grades:

- Grade 1 (Mild): Transient confusion without loss of consciousness, and symptoms resolve in <15 minutes.
- Grade 2 (Moderate): Transient confusion without loss of consciousness, and symptoms resolve in >15 minutes.
- Grade 3 (Severe): Any loss of consciousness of any duration.

18. A: Because the most common reason for a fall in CVP is hypovolemia, a rapid fluid infusion of 250 to 500 mL may be given. If the pressure again starts to fall ≤10 minutes, then the fall indicates probable hypovolemia. Serial readings should always be used to verify increase or decrease. CVP is the pressure in the superior vena cava near the right atrium and helps to evaluate the function of the right atrium and right ventricle and the flow of blood back into the heart. Normal ranges for CVP are 0 to 8 cm H_2O or 2 to 6 mm Hg (depending on the type of measurement used).

19. B: The primary indications of mandibular fracture include malocclusion and ecchymosis of the floor of the mouth. An interdental gap may be evident. Most injuries result from blunt trauma, and multiple fractures may be present. Hemorrhage is uncommon with blunt injuries although bleeding may occur if the fracture lacerates an artery, such as the inferior alveolar artery; however, surgical exploration is rarely necessary as fracture reduction, application of pressure, and/or local anesthetic with epinephrine are usually sufficient to control bleeding.

20. D: Severe increasing pain that is unrelieved by analgesia and located distal to the injury (in this case, the forearm) is an initial sign of compartment syndrome, which is usually caused by bleeding into the tissue. On examination, the compartment feels tense and pain may be present with passive stretching of the muscles. Patients may develop paraesthesia and hypoaesthesia. Motor weakness is a late sign as is vascular insufficiency, so the nurse should not assume that finding a pulse below the injury precludes compartment syndrome.

21. C: Heat is generated during the drying process of a cast, so the feeling of the cast being hot and uncomfortable is normal. The patient should be advised to be sure to keep the cast uncovered until it is completely dry (24 to 48 hours). The limb should be kept elevated to decrease swelling but may be supported on a pillow, which may help prevent the cast becoming misshapen as it dries. The patient should be turned every 2 hours to allow air to circulate about the cast so that it dries evenly.

22. B: Management of umbilical cord prolapse includes elevating the presenting part off the cord, having the mother elevate her knees to the chest, and preparing for C-section. A prolapse of the umbilical cord occurs when the umbilical cord precedes the fetus in the birth canal and becomes entrapped by the descending fetus. An occult cord prolapse occurs when the umbilical cord is beside or just ahead of the fetal head. About half of prolapses occur in the second stage of labor and relate to premature delivery, multiple gestation, polyhydramnios, breech delivery, and an excessively long umbilical cord.

23. A: When assessing the ABCDEs (Airway, Breath/ventilation, Circulation, Disability, Exposure/environmental control) of a patient with a traumatic brain injury, indications of Cushing's triad (bradycardia, hypertension, and abnormal irregular respirations) may be a sign of brainstem herniation. Herniation most often results from increasing intracranial pressure that interferes with blood flow to the brain and oxygenation.

24. A: A patient with blunt trauma to the lower jaw and suspected mandibular fracture should first be assessed for airway obstruction, which may result from avulsed teeth lodging in the airway or bilateral fractures. The patient should have the head elevated and oral suctioning carried out if necessary. The anterior flail portions of the fractured mandible may be manually positioned anteriorly to open the airway temporarily.

25. C: Defusing sessions usually occur very early, sometimes during a stressful event, and are used to educate personnel about what to expect over the next few days and to provide guidance in handling feelings and stress. Debriefing sessions usually follow in one to three days and may be repeated periodically as needed. People are encouraged to express their feelings and emotions about the event. Critiquing the event or attempting to place blame is not productive as part of the CISM process.

26. B: The fundus should be firm and midline. A deviation to one side or the other is often related to bladder distention, so this should be evaluated and the mother offered a bedpan or allowed to use a toilet if possible. If unable to urinate, she may need to be catheterized. Hemorrhage results in a boggy, soft fundus. Uterine rupture usually occurs during labor and is associated with pain, bleeding, and signs of shock.

27. D: PVCs or increase in the amplitude of the T waves is consistent with irritation of the epicardium from contact with the needle, so the needle should be slowly withdrawn until the PVCs stop and the ECG returns to baseline readings. Acute injury to the myocardium may elicit changes in the ST segment or QRS complex. A laceration of the peritoneum may not be evident at the time of injury but may result in subsequent infection and peritonitis. Other injuries can include damage to coronary arteries or veins, pneumothorax, esophageal laceration, and pneumopericardium.

28. C: A patient with a basilar skull fracture is especially at risk of cerebrospinal fluid leakage (occurring in about 20%) because these fractures often involve the petrous temporal bone (70%). CSF may leak from the nose or ear. Diagnosis of CSF leak can be difficult because glucose tests are unreliable. Beta2-transferrin testing is most accurate but not widely available. High-resolution CTs may help to identify defects that can cause leakage.

29. C: A complete physical examination is done as part of the secondary survey, including a neurological assessment. The ATLS protocol steps include:

- Primary survey: Assessment of ABCs (airway, breathing, and circulation).
- Resuscitation: Active efforts to resuscitate and stabilize patient.
- Secondary survey: Reviews the ABCs and adds DE to the original—disability and exposure/examination to provide further information about the extent of injury.
- Definitive treatment: Treatment may include surgery or other medical treatment as indicated.

30. B: The "death triangle" associated with rapid resuscitation includes acidosis, coagulopathy, and hypothermia. ATLS protocol calls for 2L (crystalloid) rapid bolus for adults and 20 mL/kg for children. Transfusions may be added with extensive blood loss. Protocol calls for two large bore IVs although central line may be needed in some cases. Short tubing and compression may allow infusion rates up to 500 mL/min, but this may rapidly cool the patient. Hypothermia may increase coagulopathy, so warming IV fluids, keeping the ambient temperature at 21°C, and using warming blankets may help prevent complications.

31. D: The initial treatment for status epilepticus (SE) is a fast-acting benzodiazepine (such as Ativan®), often in steps with administration every 5 minutes until seizures subside. If there is no response to the first 2 doses of anticonvulsants (refractory SE), rapid sequence intubation (RSI), which involves sedation and paralytic anesthesia, may be done while therapy continues. Phenytoin and phenobarbitol may be added, but combining phenobarbitol and benzodiazepine can cause apnea, so intubation may be necessary. Acyclovir and ceftriaxone may be administered if cause is unknown as SE may be triggered by viral encephalitis.

32. C: If a patient who experienced facial trauma has epistaxis from tearing of posterior vessels of the nose, the most likely treatment is compression tamponade, which may be done with an inflatable Foley catheter or packing. Tearing of anterior vessels, on the other hand, is usually more easily controlled with direct pressure, cold compresses, or nasal vasoconstrictive spray. In both cases, the patient should be positioned with the head elevated.

33. A: While all of these are important, the critical assessment is of vascular status because dislocation of the knee often tears the popliteal artery. Knee dislocation places the patient at high risk of compartment syndrome and amputation, especially if circulation is impaired for more than 6 hours. The presence of pedal pulses is not sufficient to rule out vascular injury, so the patient must undergo arteriograms or ultrasound evaluation. Nerve assessment is also important, as injury to the tibial and peroneal branches of the sciatic nerve is common.

34 D: The date of the last tetanus shot is especially important for all open contaminated wounds. Patients whose tetanus toxoid injections are up-to-date and have had three or more immunizations generally require no further preventive treatment; however, if the patient is not immunized, has had fewer than three immunizations, or is unclear about immunization, then the patient should receive both the tetanus toxoid and tetanus immune globulin because tetanus toxoid does not confer immediate immunity while tetanus immune globulin provides temporary immunity immediately.

35. D: Risk of FES is greatest with multiple fractures or fractures of long bones, ribs, or pelvis. Those 20-30 years and elderly adults with fracture of proximal femur are at increased risk. Onset of symptoms (hypoxia, tachypnea, elevated temperature, and tachycardia) is usually at 24 to 72 hours but may be delayed for up to 7 days:

- Early signs include respiratory alkalosis progressing to respiratory acidosis, leading to respiratory distress syndrome and congestive heart failure.
- Fat emboli in the brain cause CNS abnormalities, such as headache and confusion leading to coma.
- Systemic embolization may cause widespread petechiae, elevated temperature (>39.5°C), and kidney failure.

36. C: For a patient with contained blunt aortic injury but multiple other injuries that require delay in surgical repair, antihypertensives are administered to maintain systolic blood pressure below 120 mm Hg to reduce the stress on the injured area. While almost always requiring surgical repair, repair of contained injuries may need to be delayed if the patient has other severe injuries, such as head injuries, pulmonary injuries, or coagulopathy. The proximal descending aorta is the most commonly injured with blunt thoracic trauma and should always be suspected because clinical signs may be absent, especially if the aorta has a partial-thickness tear.

37. D: Because bones are very vascular, a fracture may result in hemorrhage (internal or external), especially if blood loss is substantial immediately after the fracture occurs. The patient is at greatest risk if fractures occur in the long bones, especially the femur. Other fractures that pose risk of hypovolemic shock include fractures of the pelvis, thorax, and vertebrae. Patients with any type of major fracture should be monitored carefully to observe for signs of hypovolemic shock.

38. A: If an adult patient has second- and third-degree burns of both arms (front and back) (9 + 9 = 18), the front of the trunk (18) and the perineum (1), the total body surface area (TBSA) that is burned is 37% (18 +18 +1 = 37). Rule of 9s estimates BSA burned: <u>Adults</u>—9% head, trunk (front) 18%, trunk (back) 18%, arm 9%, leg 18%, perineum 1%. <u>Infants/Children</u>—18% head, trunk (front) 185, trunk (back) 18%, arm 9%, leg 14%, perineum 1%.

39. D: Muscle spasms are a common complaint of those with fractured vertebrae, and the treatment that may provide the most relief is to apply heat to the fractured area as this improves circulation and relaxes the muscles. Pain increases on movement and weight bearing. Patient may also be prescribed muscle relaxants to help alleviate muscle spasms. Unstable fractures usually require immediate surgery to prevent further neurological deficits; however, stable fractures can usually be treated conservatively.

40. C: If a patient has small shards of glass lodged in the surface of both corneas, after instillation of a topical anesthetic, the foreign bodies are usually removed with a 21-gauge needle, gently dislodging and removing them one at a time under slit-lamp magnification. If shards are imbedded deeply, then surgical removal may be necessary. Patients with corneal foreign bodies typically have pain and tearing and may feel as though something is in the eye. Following removal, antibiotic ophthalmic ointment is applied and the eye patched.

41. B: The most common traumatic intracerebral lesion is the subdural hematoma and is found in almost a third of patients with head injuries, so it should always be suspected. If present, there may also be underlying injuries. Acute subdural hematomas occur in fewer than 72 hours after injury while subacute occur up to 7 days after injury and chronic 21 days or more after injury. The treatment of choice is generally surgical evacuation.

42. D: About 33 percent of those with unstable pelvic fractures has injury to the urethra, so before a Foley catheter is inserted into the bladder, a retrograde urethrogram should be completed. Other tests, such as a cystogram or intravenous pyelogram may be ordered if indicated. Unstable fractures also put the patient at increased risk of hemorrhage and various other internal injuries, so a thorough examination of the perineal area and a rectal exam should also be completed before catheter placement.

43. A: The first step to applying a TLSO brace is for the patient to put on a tight-fitting t-shirt to protect the skin and prevent chafing. Next, the patient puts the arm through the opening that lies between the shoulder strap and the lumbar portion on one side. The metal sternal attachment is then centered and the lumbar belt pulled around and fastened. Then, the shoulder strap on the other side is attached through the loop on the sternal bar. The metal bar of the sternal attachment should be 4 finger-widths below the sternal notch. Last, the straps on the lumbar portion are tightened and attached.

44. A: The cauda equina is the group of nerves at the end of the spinal cord, containing the nerve roots for L1 to S5 vertebrae. Compression of the nerves of the cauda equina, most often occurring at L4 and L5, can result in cauda equina syndrome, which presents as "saddle" numbness of the buttocks and lower legs. The legs may become progressively weak and the patient may experience fecal and urinary incontinence and impotence. Surgical decompression of the nerves must be done immediately to prevent permanent damage.

45. B: Gross negligence would be indicated in this scenario. Negligence indicates that *proper care* has not been provided, based on established standards. *Reasonable care* uses rationale for decision-making in relation to providing care. Types of negligence include:

- <u>Negligent conduct</u> indicates that an individual failed to provide reasonable care or to protect/assist another, based on standards and expertise.
- <u>Gross negligence</u> is willfully providing inadequate care while disregarding the safety and security of another.
- Contributory negligence involves the injured party contributing to his or her own harm.
- <u>Comparative negligence</u> attempts to determine what percentage amount of negligence is attributed to each individual involved.

46. C: Underlying injuries should be expected according to the area of fractures:

- Upper 2 ribs: Injuries to trachea, bronchi, or great vessels.
- Right-sided ≥rib 8: Trauma to liver.
- Left-sided ≥ rib 8: Trauma to spleen.

Pain, often localized or experienced on respirations or compression of chest way may be the primary symptom of rib fractures, resulting in shallow breathing that can lead to atelectasis or pneumonia. Fractured ribs are usually the result of severe trauma, such as blunt force from a motor vehicle accident or physical abuse.

47. D: <u>Autonomy</u> is the ethical principle that the individual has the right to make decisions about his or her own care. The nurse practitioner must keep the patients fully informed so they can exercise autonomy in informed decision-making. <u>Beneficence</u> is an ethical principle that involves performing actions that are for the purpose of benefitting another person. <u>Nonmaleficence</u> is an ethical principle that means healthcare workers should provide care in a manner that does not cause direct intentional harm to the patient. <u>Justice</u> is the ethical principle that relates to the distribution of the limited resources of healthcare benefits to the members of society.

48. B: Beck's triad is an indication of cardiac tamponade, treated with pericardiocentesis with large bore needle or surgical repair to control bleeding and relieve cardiac compression. Cardiac tamponade occurs with pericardial effusion in which fluid accumulates in the pericardial sac, causing pressure against the heart. It may be a complication of trauma, pericarditis, cardiac surgery, or heart failure. Other symptoms may include a feeling of pressure or pain in the chest as well as dyspnea, and pulsus paradoxus >10 mm Hg (systolic blood pressure heard during exhalation but not during inhalation).

49. A: If a patient is suspected of having compartment syndrome associated with abdominal trauma and shock, intraabdominal pressure is usually assessed by inserting a Foley catheter attached to a pressure transducer into the empty bladder. The catheter is clamped and transducer zeroed at the iliac crest along the midaxillary line. Then, about 10 mL (2 to 25 mL) of fluid is injected into the bladder and left in place for 30-60 seconds before reading the pressure following a patient expiration. Compartment pressures should be <30 mm Hg and the difference between diastolic BP and compartment pressure should be >30 mm Hg.

50. D: Patients who receive multiple transfusions with citrated blood products must be carefully monitored for hypocalcemia. Calcium is important for transmitting nerve impulses and regulating muscle contraction and relaxation, including the myocardium. Calcium activates enzymes that stimulate chemical reactions and has a role in coagulation of blood. Values include:

- Normal values: 8.2 to 10.2 mg/dL.
- Hypocalcemia: <8.2 mg/dL. Critical value: <7 mg/dL.
- Hypercalcemia: >10.2 mg/dL. Critical value: >12 mg/dL.

Symptoms include tetany, tingling, seizures, altered mental status, and ventricular tachycardia. Treatment is calcium replacement and vitamin D.

51. C: Wounds should be irrigated with pressures of 10 to 15 psi. An irrigation pressure of <4 psi does not adequately cleanse a wound, and pressures >15 psi can result in trauma to the wound, interfering with healing. A mechanical irrigation device is more effective for irrigation than a bulb syringe, which delivers about ≤2 psi. A 250 mL squeeze bottle supplies about 4.5 psi, adequate for low-pressure cleaning. A 35-mL syringe with a 19-gauge needle provides about 8 psi.

52. A: These symptoms are consistent with fat embolism syndrome (FES), which may cause rapid acute pulmonary edema and ARDS, so the patient should be immediately provided with high-flow oxygen. Controlled-volume ventilation with PEEP may be indicated to prevent/treat pulmonary edema. Corticosteroids may reduce inflammation of the lungs and reduce cerebral edema. Vasopressors prevent hypotension and interstitial pulmonary edema. Morphine with a benzodiazepine may be indicated for patients who require artificial ventilation.

53. B: EMTALA prohibits patient "dumping" from EDs. Stabilization of emergent conditions or active labor must be done prior to transfer, and the patient's condition should not deteriorate during transfer. HIPAA addresses the rights of the individual related to privacy of health information. ADA is civil rights legislation that provides the disabled, including those with mental impairment, access to employment and the community. OAA provides improved access to services for older adults and Native Americans, including community services (meals, transportation, home health care, adult day care, legal assistance, and home repair).

54. A: Child Protective Services should be notified so authorities can investigate the possibility of child abuse. Spiral fractures of the shafts of long bones are the most common abuse-related fracture in children. Additionally, new bruises should be red-purple. Widespread yellow-green and brown bruises suggest earlier injuries. A 3-year old child is not a reliable reporter, and forewarning the parent by questioning him or her about abuse or giving advice may cause an abusive parent to remove the child from care to avoid detection.

55. D: The best solution is a referral to a home health agency to provide in-home care, as this ensures that the woman will receive skilled nursing care and be able to stay at home and supervise her granddaughter. A 12-year old is too young for the responsibility of wound care. The patient's dependence on public transportation and difficulty walking precludes outpatient care. Home health care is a more cost-effective solution than transferring the patient to an extended care facility, which would leave the granddaughter without care. Medicare will not pay for extended hospital care for healing wounds.

56. C: I and IV. If a blood specimen is obtained from a patient with a suspected highly infectious pathogen, the case should be discussed with the laboratory personnel prior to collection to ensure that proper procedures are followed, and the laboratory should be notified in advance so that they can take extra precautions as indicated. Protocols should be utilized for preparation and transport. Highly infectious pathogens include ebola virus, *Mycobacterium tuberculosis, N. meningitidis, Francisella tularensis,* SARS coronavirus, and H5N1.

57. C: Ideally, patients on droplet precautions should be maintained in private rooms or cohorted with another patient infected with the same organism (but no other infection). However, if these options are not available, the patient may be placed in a room with a non-infected patient with a spatial separation of at least 3 feet and a curtain between them. The door may be kept open and no special air handling is required. Patient transport should be limited.

58. A: If a patient with inhalation injury has a carboxyhemoglobin (COHB) level completed with initial lab work as part of evaluation for carbon monoxide poisoning, a normal percentage of COHB is less than 5%. If the level is ≥20%, patients are usually asymptomatic, but at 20% to 30%, patients exhibit headache, impairment of fine muscle control, nausea, and vomiting. At 30% to 40%, patients become weak and lethargic. At 40% to 50%, patients lapse into comas, and death occurs with levels greater than 60%.

59. D: The most common type of transmission of infectious organisms in the healthcare facility is contact transmission, especially associated with inadequate hand washing. Healthcare personnel may be less susceptible to infection than patients who are ill, so the healthcare personnel can become colonized, such as with nasal *Staphylococcus aureus,* and serve as carriers. If personnel don't wash their hands after caring for a patient, they can carry bacteria directly on their skin from one patient to another.

60. C: If a patient receiving packed red blood cells develops febrile nonhemolytic reaction (NHR) with chills, fever, headache, muscle ache, restlessness, and flushing, but BP and respiratory status remain stable, the reaction the patient is having is probably directed at the residual white blood cells. The transfusion can usually be resumed after the patient is administered antipyretics. If a patient has a history of NHR, then leukocyte-depleted RBCs may be indicated.

61. B: If prehospital, a patient is found lying on the street with multiple stab wounds and the knife protruding from the right chest, during transport, the knife should be padded for support about the handle and any protruding shaft as removing it may result in severe hemorrhage. Holding the knife in place manually increases risk that the knife may be jarred during transport.

62. D: According to CDC guidelines, in the emergency response to a needlestick or a cut, the first action is to wash the area with soap and water. Splashes of body fluids or contaminated liquids to the face, skin, mouth, or nose should be flushed with water and eyes irrigated with normal saline, clean water, or sterile irrigant. Following this emergency step, the incident should be immediately reported to a supervisor and medical treatment sought to determine if post-exposure prophylaxis is indicated.

63. A: Rankings may be calculated with various measures, including raw scores and mean/average scores, but for comparison purposes, when looking at benchmarks, percentile ranking is often utilized. A score of 69% indicates that this unit scored better than 69% of those the unit was benchmarking against.

Score may be classified as being in the top decile (10%) or quartile (25%) as well. The goal is generally to score at least at the 50% ranking and to steadily increase percentile rankings.

64. D: I, II, III, and IV. When developing a plan to respond to acts of terrorism involving release of biologic agents, necessary components include a developing a phone/email tree to notify all necessary staff and public health officials; stockpiling of adequate personal protective equipment and respirators; developing procedures for handling of deaths; developing procedures for monitoring for air and water contamination; assigning staff to serve as liaisons among different agencies; accommodating large numbers of new patients with contact, droplet, and/or airborne precautions; training staff; and educating the public about signs, symptoms, and preventive measures.

65. D: A gunshot wound to the intraperitoneal area of the abdomen increases risk of injury to the liver and spleen. Other organs at risk include hollow organs, such as the stomach, parts of the small intestine (ileum, jejunum), the descending portion of the colon, the rectum, and primary vessels of the abdomen. Gunshot wounds to the retroperitoneal area increase risk of injury to organs of the urinary system, pancreas, rectum, and colon (ascending and descending) as well as to primary vessels of the abdomen.

66. B: When instructing families and visitors about methods to prevent and control infections, the best approach is to focus on their using proper hand hygiene before and after patient contact. Because contact transmission is the most common type of transmission, hand washing is the best and easiest defense. While posters and literature about infection control may be helpful, many people are oblivious to them or fail to read them fully. Unless patients are on isolation, there are usually no restrictions about proximity or touching environmental surfaces.

67. D: <u>Onset of symptoms:</u> Note how and when the symptoms started and any contributing factors, including a review of treatments. <u>Degree of deformity:</u> Evaluate pain, swelling, stiffness and reports of limitations. Observe for changes, such as enlarged joints. <u>Paralysis/Paresis:</u> Note onset and extent and any changes, such as regression or progression of symptoms. <u>Pain:</u> Note the type of pain, where it's located, the severity, duration, any contributing or precipitating factors, and any other symptoms associated with the pain (such as increased weakness).

68. A: These blood gas changes indicate the patient is experiencing acute respiratory acidosis, which is characterized by an increase of 10 mm Hg in $PaCO_2$ resulting in a decrease of 0.08 in pH. In chronic respiratory acidosis, the pH decreases by 0.03. Normal blood gas values include:

- Acidity/alkalinity (pH): 7.35-7.45.
- Partial pressure of carbon dioxide ($PaCO_2$): 35-45 mm Hg.
- Partial pressure of oxygen (PaO_2): ≥80 mg Hg.
- Bicarbonate concentration (HCO_3): 22-26 mEq/L.
- Oxygen saturation (SaO_2): ≥95%.

69. B: If SPO_2 falls, the oximeter should be repositioned, as incorrect position is a common cause of inaccurate readings. The oximeter uses light waves to determine oxygen saturation (SPO_2). Pulse oximetry, continuous or intermittent, utilizes an external oximeter that attaches to the patient's finger or earlobe to measure arterial oxygen saturation (SPO_2), the percentage of hemoglobin that is saturated with oxygen. Oxygen saturation should be maintained >95% although some patients with chronic respiratory disorders, such as COPD may have lower SPO_2. Results may be compromised by impaired circulation, excessive light, poor positioning, and nail polish.

70. C: If patients have difficulty coordinating inhalation and actuation of the inhaler (a common problem) after repeated attempts, then the best solution is often for the patient to use a different delivery system or an adapter, such as the Autohaler® actuator, or a reservoir device, which contains a holding chamber for the aerosol. Studies show that over half of patients use MDIs incorrectly, affecting dosage of medication so ensuring that patients are able to correctly use inhalers is critical.

71. A: The "talk and die" phenomenon in which a patient loses consciousness after a blow to the head and then recovers and appears to be fine before suddenly developing severe symptoms of brain injury is typical of epidural hemorrhage, which is bleeding between the skull and the dura mater, resulting in compression of the underlying brain tissue. With rapid treatment, prognosis is good, but if the lesion expands rapidly, a midline shift and herniation may occur.

72. B: If 15 hours after a patient was involved in an automobile accident, the patient presents in the trauma center with abdominal discomfort and a positive Cullen's sign (bruising about the umbilicus), the trauma nurse should suspect retroperitoneal bleeding or hemoperitoneum. This sign is usually not evident for about 12 hours. Other indications include a positive Grey Turner's sign (bruising over flank). The patient may also have hematuria and hemodynamic instability.

73. D: The most common cause of distributive shock is sepsis (septic shock). With distributive shock, arterial/venous dilation occurs, resulting in decreased systemic vascular resistance and decreased cardiac output and tissue hypoperfusion although blood volume is normal. Sepsis usually develops from bacteremia. Common causes include *E. coli, Klebsiella, Proteus,* and *Pseudomonas.* Risk factors include older age, diabetes, recent invasive procedures, and immunosuppression. Distributive shock may occur with sepsis, anaphylaxis, neurological insult, vasodilator drugs, and acute adrenal insufficiency.

74. C: Systemic inflammatory response syndrome (SIRS) is characterized by at least two indications, which may include:

- Elevated (>38°C) or subnormal rectal temperature (<36°C).
- Tachypnea or $PaCO_2$ <32 mm Hg.
- Tachycardia.
- Leukocytosis (>12,000) or leukopenia (<4000).

SIRS, a generalized inflammatory response affecting may organ systems, may be caused by infectious or non-infectious agents, such as trauma, burns, adrenal insufficiency, pulmonary embolism, and drug overdose. If an infectious agent is identified or suspected, SIRS is an aspect of sepsis.

75. B: If a patient is brought to the trauma center after a motorcycle accident and exhibits bruising over the area of the mastoid process (Battle's sign) as well as otorrhea, these are indications of a basilar skull fracture. Rhinorrhea (clear CSF) and bilateral swelling and ecchymosis of the eyes (raccoon eyes) can also indicate a basilar skull fracture. Basilar skull fractures may occur from impacts to the occipital or mandibular areas and may result in damage to the olfactory and optic nerves.

76. A: A patient with severe blunt trauma to the liver receiving fluid resuscitation during transportation to the trauma center to treat hypotension and unstable condition is especially at risk of hemorrhage (the most common complication) and hemodilution because of the combination of bleeding and fluid resuscitation. Hemorrhage may require ligation of hepatic arteries or veins. Treatment often includes intravenous fluids for fluid volume deficit as well as blood products (plasma, platelets) for coagulopathies. Liver trauma is often associated with multiple organ damage as well.

77. B: The fracture that is likely to result in the greatest loss of blood is the pelvis.

Estimated blood loss with fractures (in liters)	
Ankle	0.5 to 1.5
Elbow	0.5 to 1.5
Femur	1 to 2
Hip	1.5 to 2.5
Humerus	1 to 2
Knee	1 to 1.5
Pelvis	1.5 to 4.5
Tibia	0.5 to 1.5

78. C: Justice is the ethical principle that relates to the distribution of the limited resources of healthcare benefits to the members of society. These resources must be distributed fairly. This issue may arise if there is only one bed left and two sick patients. Justice comes into play in deciding which patient should stay and which should be transported or otherwise cared for. The decision should be made according to what is best or most just for the patients and not colored by personal bias.

79. B: Class II.

Hemorrhagic shock classification

Class	Blood loss	Signs and symptoms
I	≤15% (up to 750 mL)	Mild tachycardia (90-100 bpm), localized swelling, and frank bleeding. BP normal. Respirations 14-20. Urine: >30 mL/hr. Patient sl. anxious.
II	15 to 25% (750-1500 mL)	Tachycardia (>100), prolonged capillary refill and increased diastolic BP. Respirations 20-30. Urine 20-30 mL/hr. Patient mildly anxious.
III	25 to 50% (1500-2000 mL)	Above signs (any), tachycardia (>120) as well as hypotension, confusion, decreased urinary output, and acidosis. Respirations 30-40. Urine: 5-15 mL/hr. Patient anxious and confused.
IV	>50% (>200 mL)	Tachycardia (>140), hypotension and acidosis unresponsive to resuscitation. Respirations >35. Urine: Scant. Patient confused and lethargic.

80. A: If a patient presents in the emergency department after falling from a horse and being kicked in the left side and has a fractured left lower rib and is exhibiting elevation of the left hemidiaphragm, left lower lobe atelectasis, and pleural effusion as well as tachycardia, hypotension, left flank pain, and positive Kehr sign (pain referred to left shoulder), the trauma nurse should recognize these signs and symptoms as indications of ruptured spleen. Immediate surgical exploration may be needed to prevent the patient from bleeding out.

81. D: If a patient who was a victim of a violent assault and rape is shaking and crying and appears terrified, the most therapeutic response at the time of the initial encounter with the patient is, "You are safe now." The patient is likely still in the "fight or flight" mode with increased adrenalin from having to deal with the assault and rape, police intervention, and now a medical examination, so it's important for the trauma nurse to provide calm reassurance to the patient to try to allay fears.

82. C: Level IV. Trauma Center designations (ACS):

- Level I (highest): Complete care for all types of injuries, including 24-hour general surgeons and various specialists and can provide rehabilitation services, cardiac surgery, hemodialysis, and microsurgery.
- Level II: Less comprehensive and must transfer some patients to level I for tertiary care.
- Level III: 24-hour immediate care by physicians and surgeons/anesthesiologists promptly available. Not all subspecialties are available, but can transfer patients.
- Level IV: trauma nurse(s) and physician(s) available on patient arrival, can provide advanced life support and stabilization for transfer.
- Level V (lowest): Basic ED with trauma nurse(s) and physician(s) available on patient arrival and may provide surgery and critical-care services and transfer patients.

83. A: Total loss of respiratory muscle function occurs with spinal cord injuries above C4. The diaphragm is innervated by the phrenic nerve (C3 to C5), so injury above this level requires immediate intubation and ventilation. Even with injuries below C4, intercostal muscles may be paralyzed, resulting in hypoventilation. If abdominal muscles are paralyzed, then the patient may be unable to cough or clear the airway. Those with injuries at C5 or higher usually have a tracheostomy performed to facilitate mechanical ventilation.

84. B: The patient should remove the clothing if possible and place each piece of clothing in a separate paper bag, or the trauma nurse should carefully remove the clothing, taking care to avoid cutting through cuts or tears from gunshot or knife wounds. The nurse should wear disposable gloves when handling clothing gently so that evidence, such as strands of hair or other materials, is not lost in transfer. A clean sheet or drape should be placed on the floor and collection paper over that so the patient can stand on the collection paper while removing clothing if possible.

85. D: When preparing to administer a unit of packed red blood cells and the trauma nurse notes gas bubbles in the blood, this may indicate bacterial infection, so the unit should be returned to the blood center. Any abnormalities in the color of the blood (discoloration, cloudiness) may indicate hemolysis. PRBCs should be administered within one-half hour of refrigeration, and administration should not be longer than 4 hours. A blood filter should be used and changed after every second unit.

86. A: These VS changes are consistent with increasing intracranial pressure. Typical findings include widened pulse pressure, with rising blood pressure and depressed heart rate. Because the patient is drunk, evaluating level of consciousness can be difficult, but lethargy, confusion, and restlessness are characteristic of increasing ICP. Stress response usually results in increased BP and pulse. Ethanol intoxication usually causes hypotension, bradycardia with arrhythmias, and respiratory depression. Delirium tremens includes tremors, tachycardia, and cardiac dysrhythmias.

87. C: A woman in active premature labor with a singleton or multiple births ≥20 weeks gestation should be airlifted because the infant(s) may be viable. Burns require air transport if they involve explosion with respiratory distress or confusion, unconsciousness, or ≥18% (second or third degree) of BSA require air transport. Fractures can be immobilized for ground transport. Penetrating trauma (shrapnel, GSW, stabbing) to the head (especially with prolonged unconsciousness) or trunk usually requires air transport, but injury to a limb, unless associated with severe bleeding or impaired circulation, is less critical.

88. D: Patients should be offloaded ONLY when a crewmember signals the receiving medical personnel to approach the aircraft. Prior to offloading, the crew will usually shut down the aircraft, and this requires about 2 minutes. A rotor aircraft, such as the helicopter, does not require that people approach in a crouching position, but people should avoid holding anything over their heads and should generally approach from the front of the aircraft and avoid the rear of the aircraft and the rear rotors.

89. A: The pediatric BIG (bone injection gun) for intraosseous infusion is intended for use only in the proximal tibia of children from birth (term) to 12 years of age. The adult BIG injection gun for those 12 and older may be used in either the proximal tibia or proximal humerus. The pediatric BIG contains an 18-gauge needle and insertion depth can be adjusted from 0.5 to 1.5 cm, according to age. The adult BIG contains a 15-gauge needle with a preset insertion depth of 2.5 cm. FAST needles are used for IO infusions into the sternum.

90. C: If, at the site of an explosion, a patient with multiple shrapnel wounds in the left arm has severe uncontrolled bleeding, when placing a tourniquet to control bleeding during transit, the trauma nurse should place the tourniquet proximally ('high and tight") on the left extremity. With a single wound, a tourniquet may be placed high or 2 to 3 inches above the wound, but with multiple wounds and in emergent situations, the best choice is to place proximally to allow for rapid transit.

91. B: When attempting to control hemorrhage with permissive hypotension, in order to maintain adequate perfusion, the systolic blood pressure should not fall below 80 mm Hg, and the patient must be carefully monitored for signs of hypoperfusion. Protocols may vary somewhat from one institution to another and according to the situation. For example, permissive hypotension with systolic blood pressure maintained at 80-100 mg may be indicated when massive transfusion protocols are activated. Permissive hypotension decreases risk of emboli, coagulopathy, and hypothermia associated with high-dose rapid fluid resuscitation.

92. A: An indication for an open thoracotomy at bedside for a patient is loss of greater than 1500 mL of blood per chest tube. Other indications include pulselessness after witnessed cardiac activity and hypotension (systolic BP <70 mm Hg) despite resuscitation attempts. Contraindications include lack of witnessed cardiac activity, nontraumatic cardiac arrest, severe traumatic brain injury, and severe multisystem injuries. Survival rates for open thoracotomy at bedside after penetrating trauma (gunshot and stab wounds) are better than after blunt trauma.

93. D: Confirmability. In evaluating research as part of the development of evidence-based practice guidelines, the four evaluative/trustworthiness criteria are:

- Credibility: Documentation supports accuracy and validity.
- Dependability: Evidence shows how conclusions are reached and whether others should expect to each the same conclusions.
- Transferability: The extent to which the results can apply to others in similar situations.
- Confirmability: The data are clear and show how conclusions are reached.

94. C: A primary consideration of mortality and morbidity reviews is improvement in the provision of care. MMRs are confidential to encourage free and open discussion of sentinel events and serious incidents/complications in order to explore exactly what happened, if standards of care were breached, where errors occurred, what was done correctly, why the event/incident/complication occurred, what steps can be taken to avoid a recurrence of this same type of problems, and what can be learned.

95. B: If a patient involved in a motorcycle accident is maintained on life support but meets the criteria for brain death and does not carry an organ donor card, the trauma nurse's responsibility is generally to ensure the organ procurement organization is notified. Families are generally approached by OPO representatives or trained staff rather than trauma personnel (while the patient remains on life support) to ask for permission to obtain organs and tissue for donation.

96. C: "The law doesn't allow me to give out any information about patients in order to protect their privacy and safety" is accurate and appropriate. The Health Insurance Portability and Accountability Act (HIPAA) addresses the privacy of health information. It is essential to never release any information or documentation about a client's condition or treatment without consent. Personal information about the client is considered protected health information (PHI), and it includes any identifying or personal information about the client, such as health history, condition, or treatments in any form, and any documentation. Failure to comply with HIPAA regulations can make one liable for legal action.

97. A: If a pregnant patient was involved in an automobile accident with abdominal trauma and experienced placental abruption, the patient must be carefully monitored for indications of disseminated intravascular coagulopathy (DIC). When placental abruption occurs, thromboplastin release may occur along with amniotic fluid embolus, and these in turn can result in DIC. Immediate Cesarean, evacuation of the uterus, and therapy with blood components (platelets/coagulation factors) are essential to prevent maternal mortality.

98. B: If a patient that suffered severe chest trauma result in fractured lower ribs is exhibiting hemidiaphragmatic elevation and atelectasis of the lower lobe of the left lung, this suggests diaphragmatic injury. In up to 80% of cases, diaphragmatic injuries are on the left side and are often associated with other abdominal injuries. Diagnosis is usually confirmed during laparotomy to repair tears because imaging and other tests are often inconclusive. Penetrating injuries tend to be smaller initial, but then enlarge.

99. C: The primary focus when instituting change should be on finding and utilizing the best available evidence-based research. However, the trauma nurse should also consider the expertise of those involved, such as physicians, nurses, the resources (financial, social, psychological) that are available, the characteristics of those involved, the environment, the organizational structure, the mission and values of the institution, and the impact any changes will have on those affected by the changes, such as staff, administration, and students.

100. B: If a patient is brought to the trauma center after an automobile accident with multiple fractured ribs and exhibits labored breathing with respiratory rate of 40/min and oxygen saturation of 86% and the patient is hemodynamically unstable, the trauma nurse should prepare the patient for intubation and mechanical ventilation. The patient's presentation is consistent with flail chest, and intubation is indicated with shock and/or respiratory distress, including labored breathing, respiration >35 or <8 per minute, oxygen saturation <90%, PaO_2 <60 mm Hg, and $PaCO_2$ >55 mm Hg.

101. A: An amputated body part, such as a hand, should have jewelry removed and be thoroughly irrigated to remove debris, wrapped with saline moistened dressing and placed inside a sealed plastic bag that is then immersed in ice water (1:1 ice to water). It's important to keep the part cool but to avoid freezing. The part should be reattached within 6 hours if possible but may be delayed up to 24 hours if the part is properly stored.

102. C: If a patient experienced a high voltage electrical shock with electrical burns from touching a live wire with the palm of his hand while standing and bending over, the trauma nurse would expect exit wounds at multiple sites as the current's pathway is unpredictable. With low voltage electrical shocks, the exit wound is usually at a grounded site with lowest resistance. High voltage injuries may result in severe burns, myonecrosis, thrombosis, compartment syndrome, and nerve entrapment syndrome.

103. D: If extended focused abdominal sonography for trauma (eFAST) is being used to identify pneumothorax or hemothorax associated with blunt trauma, the probe should be placed at the second intercostal space at the mid-clavicular line. Both left and right sides should be examined. FAST is a non-invasive ultrasound procedure that is part of the ATLS protocol for assessment of trauma and is generally now used in place of peritoneal lavage to detect free fluid. FAST is about 85% to 90% effective in diagnosing intraperitoneal bleeding as well as pneumo- and hemothorax and pericardial effusion.

104. B: When placing an arterial line for a patient with hemodynamic instability, the preferred access site is the radial artery with the femoral artery the second choice. Prior to insertion, adequate perfusion must be assessed and patient properly positioned:

- Radial: Perform modified Allen test, and position wrist in dorsiflexion with armboard.
- Femoral: Place patient in supine position with leg on insertion side slightly abducted and extended.

Other indications for an arterial line include frequent ABG monitoring, placement of IABP, monitoring arterial pressure, and medication administration when venous access cannot be obtained. Sterile technique is utilized for arterial line insertion.

105. C: When applying a pelvic stabilization device for a patient with a fractured pelvis, the circumferential pressure should be applied to the greater trochanter region. The pressure should be firm enough to reduce bleeding and pain, prevent further injury, and help to align the fractured areas but not so tight as to cause the fractures to overlap. Specially designed pelvic stabilization devices, such as the SAM pelvic sling, provide better support than improvised devices, such as the sheet wrap.

106. D: If using the ask-tell-ask framework to educate a patient about self-care, the trauma nurse would begin by asking the patient what the patient already knows about the condition and needs and what the patient wants to know. When the patient responds, the trauma nurse tells the patient the information needed or wanted and then asks if the patient still has more questions or needs more information, continuing the cycle of ask-tell-ask.

107. B: The 5 key elements of pain assessment include:

- Words: Used to describe pain, such as burning, stabbing, deep, shooting, and sharp. Some may complain of pressure, squeezing, and discomfort rather than pain.
- Intensity: Use of 0-10 scale or other appropriate scale to quantify the degree of pain.
- Location: Where patient indicates pain is located.
- Duration: Constant or comes and goes, breakthrough pain.
- Aggravating/alleviating factors: Those things that increase the intensity of pain and those that relieve the pain.

108. C: If a patient was raised Catholic but has not attended Mass for 50 years and is nearing death but remains responsive, the trauma nurse should ask the patient directly if the patient wants to see a priest. Even lapsed Catholics who have not been active in the church may obtain spiritual comfort from the sacraments commonly referred to as last rites. The trauma nurse should never make assumptions about a patient's spirituality.

109. C: If a 26-year-old male with no advance directive suffered a traumatic brain injury that left him in a vegetative state on life support, the family member who can legally make the decision to withdraw life support is the patient's mother. If the patient were married, the wife would be first in line, followed by adult children, parents, and then siblings. Unless the fiancée has power of attorney, the person is unrelated and, like the friend, has no legal authority to make decisions for the patient.

110. D: If a patient with blunt trauma to the genitals resulting from a physical assault has a fractured penis with gross hematosis, the trauma nurse should prepare the patient for retrograde urethrogram

170

(RUG). When a male patient experiences trauma to the genital area, such as a penile fracture, gross hematuria or evidence of blood about at the urethral meatus are indications of possible damage to the urethra. With an RUG, contrast is instilled per urethra.

111. B: If a patient with a blunt trauma neck injury has apparent laryngeal damage with subcutaneous emphysema and irregular contour of thyroid cartilage, and the patient is sitting in tripod position to ease respiratory distress, the trauma nurse should anticipate that the airway will be secured by emergent surgical airway. Any attempt to insert an oral or nasal tube may result in further damage and complete obstruction.

112. A: Underlying injuries should be expected according to the area of fractures:

- Upper 2 ribs: Injuries to trachea, bronchi, or great vessels.
- Right-sided ≥rib 8: Trauma to liver.
- Left-sided ≥ rib 8: Trauma to spleen.

Pain, often localized or experienced on respirations or compression of chest way may be the primary symptom of rib fractures, resulting in shallow breathing that can lead to atelectasis or pneumonia. Fractured ribs are usually the result of severe trauma, such as blunt force from a motor vehicle accident or physical abuse.

113. D: Staff compliance with best practice guidelines is usually best initially with simple changes in procedures, such as instituting checklists, because the learning curve is rapid and results are generally easily quantified. Because there is no financial outlay for new equipment or need for extensive training, setting up a pilot program is fairly simple. The trauma nurse should provide strong evidence based on research that the new practice is effective and should disseminate the results of a pilot program.

114. B: If a patient with a traumatic chest injury and multiple fractured ribs has shown increasing evidence of mild to moderate pulmonary contusion with slowly increasing hypoxemia and hemoptysis, the goal of fluid resuscitation in the presence of pulmonary contusion is euvolemia. Because fluid is filling the lung already, there is concern that fluid resuscitation may worsen contusion; however, the effects of hypovolemia can be life threatening, so the patient must be carefully monitored.

115. C: When checking compartment pressure in the volar compartment of the forearm using the Stryker Intracompartmental pressure monitor device, the pressure reading that indicates onset of compartment syndrome is >30 mm Hg. When the pressure is>30 mm Hg, a fasciotomy is usually needed to preserve the limb. The 5 Ps associated with compartment pressure include: pain out of proportion to injury, paresthesia, pallor, paresis, and pulse deficit.

116. B: Massive transfusion protocol (MTP) is usually activated if a patient's anticipated use of PRBCs is ≥4 units in <4 hours (although protocols may vary somewhat) or ≥10 units in 24 hours. Some patients may require up to 30 units in 8 hours. Autotransfusion may be used when appropriate. Upon activation of the protocol, the blood bank releases the MTP pack, which may vary but typically includes 4 units PRBCs, 4 units FFP, and 1 unit (6-pack) of platelets. More packs are released every 20 minutes or as needed.

117. A: A severe myocardial infarction would be excluded from a trauma registry. Trauma registries maintain records of severe traumatic injuries, such as those associated with falls, motor vehicle accidents, physical attacks, stabbings, and shootings. All level I trauma centers are required by the ACSs to maintain a trauma registry. Data elements vary but may include specific demographic information, diagnosis, treatment, stages (when appropriate), status codes, abbreviated injury scale (AIS), injury severity scale (ISS), and functional status.

118. C: The governmental agency that provides safety standards for the workplace and works is the Occupational Safety and Health Administration (OSHA). OSHA covers most employers in the private sector, but state and federal safety regulations also generally conform to OSHA standards. Employers must provide safety training, must inform workers of chemical hazards, and must provide required personal protective equipment. OSHA must be notified of a workplace-related death within 8 hour and workplace-related injury that results in hospitalization, loss of eye, or amputation within 24 hours.

119. D: If a patient has ingested sodium hydroxide, the immediate response after airway patency should be to administer one-half to one cup of milk or water to dilute it. If the patient has chemical burns on the skin, contaminated clothing should be removed and the skin flushed with copious amounts of water. Chemical burns may result from acid or alkali substances with alkali burns usually more severe than acid burns. Symptoms vary depending on the substance, strength, and site of injury but often includes severe pain, tissue blistering and sloughing, and bleeding.

120. B: If a patient with spinal cord injury at T4 has developed bradycardia, hypotension, and autonomic instability, these indications suggest the patient is developing neurogenic shock, which is a risk for those with injuries above T6. Initial treatment is rapid fluid administration of crystalloid solution to keep mean arterial pressure at 85-90 mm Hg. If hypotension persists, then inotropic agents, such as dopamine or dobutamine, may be required and atropine for persistent bradycardia.

121. A: A patient with septic shock has progressed to multi-organ dysfunction syndrome (MODS) and has developed thrombocytopenia, increasing the patient's risk of disseminated intravascular coagulation, which occurs in approximately 30% of those affected by MODS. MODS is a progression of SIRS with addition of a documented infection, organ dysfunction, hypotension, and hypoperfusion. MODS is the most common cause of sepsis-related death. Indications include depressed cardiac function, acute respiratory distress syndrome, renal failure, hepatic damage, and bowel necrosis.

122. D: If a patient with a soft tissue infection of the foot that occurred following an accidental cut has developed severe pain, erythema, tense edema, and crepitus as well as hypotension, tachycardia, and elevated temperature, the most critical emergent treatment is surgical debridement. These indications are consistent with necrotizing soft tissue infection. In some cases, multiple surgical debridements and even amputation may be required. The infection can spread rapidly and the risk of death increases markedly if surgery is delayed beyond 24 hours.

123. C: If an Rh- patient who is 7 months pregnant is involved in an automobile accident and experienced blunt abdominal trauma from the abdomen hitting the steering wheel, but the fetus does not appear to be in stress and the mother's injuries are minor although the mother has experienced some mild irregular contractions, the patient should be administered Rh-immune globulin. All Rh- pregnant patients who experience abdominal trauma or other significant trauma should automatically receive 300 mcg of Rh-immune globulin plus additional 300 mcg for every estimated 30 mL of fetal blood circulating in the maternal blood.

124. B: If a patient with a fractured pelvis from blunt trauma has gross hematuria and CT cystography shows an extraperitoneal rupture of the bladder, the most likely initial treatment for the bladder injury is insertion of a Foley catheter with continuous drainage. Most extraperitoneal ruptures will heal within 10 days (7-21 range) without surgical intervention. The Foley catheter may be inserted per urethra or suprapubically. Extraperitoneal ruptures comprise 80% of bladder ruptures and are often associated with pelvic fractures.

125. A: The primary purpose of using the SBAR format for hands-off when transferring a patient from the trauma center to a different department is to improve patient safety by ensuring important information is not overlooked. Format:

- Situation: Name, age, MD, diagnosis.
- Background: Brief medical history, co-morbidities, review of lab tests, current therapy, IV's, VS, pain, special needs, educational needs, discharge plans.
- Assessment: Review of systems, lines, tubes, and drains, completed tasks, needed tasks, future procedures.
- Recommendations: Review plan of care, medications, precautions (restraints, falls), treatments, wound care.

126. D: The first step in preventing falls is to carry out routine risk assessments with a valid assessment tool, such as the Morse Fall Risk Assessment. Risk factors include:

- Advanced age (>65).
- Dizziness/vertigo/postural hypotension.
- Confusion/disorientation/cognitive impairment.
- Severe pain.
- Impaired sensorium (hearing, vision).
- History of previous falls or fainting spells.

Interventions include identifying those at risk and making notation on chart and/or applying "at risk" wristband, use of side rails and bed in low position with the brakes applied to prevent rolling, patient visibility from nursing station, easily accessible call light, and sitter.

127. A: While all of these interventions are important, the intervention that is most likely to reduce staff injuries is a zero-lift policy because the greatest majority of nursing injuries occur when lifting, transferring, and otherwise moving patients. While avoiding all lifting may be difficult in an emergent situation, lifting must be done by appropriate numbers of staff, and transfer boards and mechanical lifting devices should be available and staff members adequately trained for use.

128. B: When beginning the chain of collection with recovery of a bullet from a gunshot wound, the three elements that must be included in addition to patient name/identifying number and signature of collecting practitioner are (1) description of item, (2) date and time of recovery, and (3) location where it was recovered. In this case, the bullet was recovered in the trauma center from the right proximal forearm, dorsal surface.

129. D: If a train crash occurs with multiple injuries and deaths and the triage team is using the black-red-yellow-green triage classification system for tagging victims, the trauma nurse would ensure the first patients to receive care are those tagged with red. Classification:

- Black: Patient is dead and will be left in the field until others are transported.
- Red: Patient is seriously injured and requires immediate attention.
- Yellow: Patient is injured but stable and can wait for transport and treatment.
- Green: "Walking wounded." Patient appears to have only minor injuries and is the lowest priority.

130. B: If a 5-year-old child cries frantically when the parents are present but quiets when the parents leave the bedside, the trauma nurse should reassure the parents that this is a normal healthy response because the child feels secure enough with the parents to express fear and anxiety through crying. If the child quiets when the parents leave the bedside, the child is probably too afraid to cry. The parents should be encouraged to assist with assessment and treatment as much as possible.

131. C: If a 16-year-old female patient is seriously injured but alert and responsive and the trauma nurse needs to find out if the patient may be pregnant but the parents are with the patient, the trauma nurse should ask the parents to step outside briefly and ask the patient in privacy. Teenagers may be reluctant to admit to being sexually active in front of parents, but all females of child-bearing age involved in trauma should be routinely asked if they may be pregnant.

132. D: IV represents a health hazard:

Irritant (to skin, eyes, and respiratory tract)	Biohazard (Body fluids)	Corrosive substances (skin burns, eye damage)	Health hazard (carcinogens, toxic substances, and respiratory irritants)

133. B: For patients with penetrating abdominal trauma, the three aspect of damage control/hemostatic resuscitation include (1) early activating of massive transfusion protocol, (2) avoiding the use of large volume crystalloid administration, and (3) utilizing permissive hypotension. For most patients with gunshot wounds, early intervention also includes abdominal laparotomy although patients with stab wounds may, in some cases, be treated more conservatively.

134. A: If a patient has second-degree burns on both hands with blistering and sloughing of outer layers of skin, the patient is likely experiencing severe pain. Initial treatment to control pain from burns generally includes an IV opioid, such as 0.1 mg/kg morphine sulfate (in titrated boluses until pain controlled). An alternative is 1.5mcg/kg intranasal fentanyl, which is also rapid acting. Once the patient's pain level is stabilized, the patient may switch to oral analgesia.

135. C: When using waveform capnography (end-tidal CO_2) to assess ventilation in a patient with a head injury, a normal finding is 35 to 45 mm Hg. Normally, when CO_2 levels increase, the body compensates by increasing respiratory rate. If the end-tidal CO_2 increases and the respiratory rate remains depressed, then the brain is not adequately managing CO_2 levels. Capnography can be used to monitor and titrate ventilation and to confirm correct placement of an endotracheal tube.

136. D: If a patient who sustained a blunt thoracic injury when hit in the chest by a hardball while playing baseball is admitted with severe chest pain, but the patient suddenly develops the following rhythm, the ECG rhythm strip represents ventricular fibrillation. The patient requires immediate defibrillation, as this is a life-threatening cardiac dysrhythmia. Ventricular fibrillation (VF) is a rapid, very irregular ventricular rate >300 beats per minute with no atrial activity observable on the ECG, caused by disorganized electrical activity in the ventricles.

137. B: If a patient experiences a distal fracture of the radius, the patient is at risk for neurovascular injury of the median nerve. The median nerve originates in the brachial plexus and runs down the length of the arm, passing through the carpal tunnel. A fracture may result in compression of the nerve and numbness and tingling in the thumb and first three fingers. Once the fracture is reduced, no further treatment is usually necessary.

138. A: With a stab wound to the abdomen, the organ that is most frequently injured is the liver (40%). For that reason, if a patient is in transit, the trauma nurse should prepare for possible severe bleeding.

Other organs at lesser risk include the small intestine, the diaphragm, and the colon. Stab wounds are more predictable than gunshot wounds with injuries usually more localized and secondary damage less likely although that may depend on the depth and trajectory of the wound.

139. C: The most effective laboratory tests when assessing oxygenation and onset of shock in a patient who is bleeding heavily are blood gases. One of the earliest signs of hypoxemia is acidotic pH (<7.25). If the level falls to 7.2, this is life-threatening metabolic acidosis. Hemoglobin and hematocrit often remain stable for the first 8 to 10 hours, and a decrease may reflect diluting effects of fluid resuscitation rather than need for transfusions. Coagulation studies may remain normal with initial bleeding.

140. D: In an unstable patient with blunt abdominal trauma, the preferred method of screening is FAST (focused assessment sonography for trauma) because it can be done quickly while the delay caused by transporting and preparing the patient for CT scan can delay critical treatment. However, for stable patients, the CT scan is generally preferred. Plain radiographs do not provide adequate information.

141. A: If a patient receiving blood transfusions shows signs of a mild allergic reaction, including pruritis, erythema, and urticaria, the usual treatment is to stop the transfusion and administer an antihistamine. Once the symptoms subside, the transfusion may be able to be restarted, but it should be administered slowly and the patient carefully monitored. If symptoms worsen, however, and the patient shows signs of shock or respiratory distress, the patient may need epinephrine, corticosteroids, and other pressor support.

142. B: Central lines may be placed into the internal jugular vein (right preferred), subclavian vein, or femoral vein (usually avoided). The right internal jugular is preferred because it has a greater diameter and better compliance than the left. Central lines allow rapid administration of large volumes of fluid, blood testing, and CVP measuring. For placement into the right jugular vein, the patient should be positioned in supine Trendelenburg position or, if not possible, with legs elevated.

143. D: If a Salem sump tube is inserted nasogastrically for a patient with bowel obstruction in order to decompress the stomach, which is painful and distended; and following insertion, the trauma nurse aspirates gastric fluids to check pH values, the value consistent with gastric fluids is 3.8. Gastric fluids tend to be very acidic (<4.0) while aspirates from the intestines are usually >4 and from the lungs, >5.5.

144. A: If a patient is involved in an accident with injury to the occipital lobe (coup injury), the other part of the brain that likely experienced injury (contrecoup) is the frontal lobes because they on the opposite side of the head and sharp edges inside the skull can cause injury. With frontal coup injuries, the occipital lobe is less likely to have damage because the inside of the skull is quite smooth in that area.

145. C: If a patient was involved in a football injury with a concussion resulting from impact to the temporal lobes, typical indications include disorientation and/or amnesia. Patients with concussion of the frontal lobes, on the other hand, are more likely to exhibit bizarre behavior. With concussion, the patient's imaging may show no signs of structure damage, but neurological functioning may be impaired for extended periods of time because of damage to neurons.

146. C: If a patient with a pneumothorax is hemodynamically stable and the physician is preparing to carry out needle decompression in the midclavicular line, the trauma nurse should prep the skin at the second and/or third intercostal space. A 10- to 14-gauge angiocath of at least 8 inches in length is used. The needle is inserted perpendicular to the skin, making sure to position the needle over the ribs instead of under where neurovascular bundles are located.

147. A: The three elements involved in establishing the mechanism of injury include:

- Questioning/Listening: Reports from the patient (if responsive and cognitively aware), family or friends, and first responders may establish how an injury occurred.
- Observation: The patient's general appearance, obvious injuries (bruises, swelling, and bleeding), and odor may provide clues.
- Physical examination: Typical patterns of injury may be associated with different mechanisms of injury.

148. B: Treatment following concussion depends on the concussion grade and includes:

- Grade 1: May return to activity within 15 minutes if no residual effects noted.
- Grade 2: May return to activity after being asymptomatic for one week for first concussion, but for second concussion, the person must have follow up with neurosurgeon and be asymptomatic for 2 weeks.
- Grade 3: The person may return to activity after follow up with neurosurgeon and be asymptomatic for 2 weeks.

149. D: It's important to approach the patient/family with full information and reasons for the transfusion or blood components without being judgmental, allowing them to express their feelings and make decisions. One should never assume that an individual would refuse blood products based on religion alone. Also, Jehovah Witnesses can receive fractionated blood cells, thus allowing hemoglobin-based blood substitutes. The following guidelines are provided to church members:

Basic blood standards for Jehovah Witnesses

Not acceptable	Whole blood: red cells, white cells, platelets, plasma
Acceptable	Fractions from red cells, white cells, platelets, and plasma

150. C: The legal document that designates someone to make decisions regarding medical and end-of-life care if a patient is mentally incompetent is a Durable Power of Attorney. This is a type of Advance Directive, which can include living wills or specific requests of the patient regarding treatment. A Do-Not-Resuscitate order indicates the patient does not want resuscitative treatment for terminal illness or condition. A General Power of Attorney allows a designated person to make decisions for a person over broader areas, including financial.

151. D: Adult patients with abdominal trauma that necessitates a splenectomy should receive the following vaccinations:

Polyvalent pneumococcal (Pneumovax 23®)	Initially and then every 6 years.
Haemophilus influenzae b conjugate (HibTITER®)	Initially, no repeat necessary.
Quadrivalent meningococcal/diphtheria conjugate (Menactra®)	Initially and then every 3 to 5 years for patients age 16 to 55.
Quadrivalent meningococcal polysaccharide (Menomune-A/C/Y/W-135®)	Initially and every 3 to 5 years for patients over age 55.

152. B: If a patient has suffered from hypothermia with reduced core temperature to 30° C, rewarming should be done slowly at the rate of 0.5 to l° C per hr. Rewarming may be carried out through infusion of warmed intravenous fluid, warm humidified air, and/or the use of warming blankets. Hypothermia occurs with exposure to low temperatures that cause the core body temperature to fall <95°F (35°C).

Autoregulation of cerebral blood flow is lost at 25° C and hypotension occurs. Deep tendon reflexes are depressed <32° C and are usually absent <26° C.

153. A: If a patient experienced a blunt impact sport-related scrotal injury and presents with severe pain and swelling of the scrotum, the trauma nurse should prepare the patient for ultrasound as it is the most effective to examine patterns of injury and blood flow to the testicles. Additionally, because urethral damage may also occur, the patient should have an RUG unless urethral damage can be ruled out. Scrotal injury may result in rupture of testis, hematocele and dislocation of the testes.

154. C: A severely mangled extremity is likely to require amputation if the score on the Mangled Extremity Severity Scoring (MESS) is greater than 7. Scores range from 1 to 14. MESS:

Category	0	1	2	3	4
Skeletal/ Soft Tissue	--	Low energy	Medium energy	High energy	Very high energy
Shock	Systolic BP >90	Transient hypotension	Persistent hypotension	--	--
Limb ischemia (Doubled if >6 hrs)	None	Mild (pulse decreased but perfusion ok)	Moderate (capillary refill decreased)	Severe capillary refill absent	--
Age	<30	30-50	>50	--	--

155. B:

Prothrombin time (PT)	10 – 15 seconds	Increases with anticoagulation therapy, vitamin K deficiency, decreased prothrombin, DIC, liver disease, and malignant neoplasm.
Partial thromboplastin time (PTT)	30 – 45 seconds	Increases with hemophilia A & B, von Willebrand's, vitamin deficiency, lupus, DIC, and liver disease.
Activated partial thromboplastin time (aPTT)	21 – 35 seconds	Similar to PTT, but decreases in extensive cancer, early DIC, and after acute hemorrhage. Used to monitor heparin dosage.
Thrombin clotting time (TCT) or Thrombin time (TT)	7 – 12 seconds (<21)	Used most often to determine dosage of heparin.
Bleeding time	2 – 9.5 minutes	Increases with DIC, leukemia, renal failure, aplastic anemia, von Willebrand's, some drugs, and alcohol.
Platelet count	150 – 400,000	Increased bleeding <50,000 and increased clotting >750,000.

156. A: A return demonstration is given by patients to show mastery of a procedure. This may be done for each step during initial instruction but should eventually include a demonstration of the entire procedure:

- The nurse should ask if the patient has any questions before the demonstration.
- The patient should gather all necessary equipment, using a checklist to ensure that nothing is forgotten.
- The patient should explain the steps.
- The nurse should provide positive feedback occasionally during the procedure: "You've placed the equipment exactly right," and may remind the patient to look at the checklist.

157. D: When assessing skeletal or soft tissue injury, a stab wound would be classified as low energy:

- Low: handgun wounds, stab wounds, simple uncomplicated fracture.
- Medium: Dislocation, multiple fractures, open fractures.
- High: Rifle gunshot wound, high speed motor vehicle accident.
- Very high: High speed trauma (such as motor vehicle accident) along with gross contamination of wound.

158. C: When carrying out the apnea test on a patient to determine brain death, the test should be aborted when the oxygen saturation falls to <90% or the patient becomes hemodynamically unstable. For the apnea test, the patient's systolic BP should be >90mm Hg with normal PaO_2 and $PaCO_2$, body temperature, and electrolytes. The patient is preoxygenated and 100% oxygen delivered per the trachea. Blood gases are measured after 5 and 10 minutes. If there is no respiratory movement and $PaCO_2$ increases to ≥60 mm Hg, the patient is brain dead. If any respiratory effort is observed, the patient is not brain dead.

159. C: Intracranial pressure monitoring is usually indicated for patients with traumatic brain injury and Glasgow Coma Score of ≥8. Uncontrolled intracranial pressure is the most common cause of mortality in neurosurgical patients and can lead to severe neurological compromise in those who survive. ICP monitoring is usually continued until the levels remain within normal range without support for 48 to 72 hours. Cerebrospinal fluid normally comprises only 5% of the volume in the skull with the brain tissues comprises 85% and blood 10%, so there is little leeway for shifts.

160. B: If a 25-year-old patient with severe neurological injury and brain death is being maintained on life support until the organs can be recovered for donation, the test that is indicated prior to organ recovery is the echocardiogram to assess the heart's function. Coronary angiograms are usually avoided in patients under 35 years. Those 35 to 45 with a history of cocaine use or greater than 3 risk factors for coronary artery disease should have coronary angiograms as well as all males over age 45 and all females over age 50.

161. D: If a nursing diagnosis for a patient with a crush injury to the right leg is "risk for ineffective tissue perfusion," an expected patient outcome to interventions is capillary refill time 3 seconds (normal 2 to 4 seconds). Additionally, the skin distal to the wound should be pink (not dusky, which indicates cyanosis) or pale. The tissue should be warm to the touch rather than cool, which suggests inadequate perfusion.

162. A: An open irregular wound resulting from the tissue tearing in response to blunt trauma is classified as a laceration. If the wound is caused by a sharp object, such as a knife or a piece of glass, it is classified as an incision. An avulsion occurs when tissue is pulled away from where it is attached or inserted. A penetration wound includes a knife wound in which the knife is inserted into the tissue and then withdrawn. A puncture wound generally retains the penetrating object, such as a nail.

163. B: If a physician has ordered negative pressure wound therapy for a patient, a contraindication to the treatment is exposed vessels because the suction applied may cause the vessels to erode and bleeding to occur. Other contraindications include malignant wounds, osteomyelitis, and non-enteric unexplored fistulae. Negative pressure wound therapy utilizes a closed system with a suction unit attached to a semi-occlusive dressing over the wound. It is especially useful for wounds that are slow healing (arterial and venous ulcers, diabetic ulcers) or that have copious discharge (non-bleeding).

164. C: A patient with extracellular fluid loss associated with bleeding is most likely to receive fluid resuscitation with isotonic IV fluid, such as normal saline (0,9% saline), 5% dextrose in water (D5W) and lactated Ringer's. Isotonic fluids may also be indicated with extracellular fluid loss related to surgery or dehydration. Because the osmolality of isotonic fluids is similar to the fluid in the human body, isotonic fluids prevent shifts of fluid from one compartment to another.

165. A: If a trauma patient needs emergent surgery but has been receiving warfarin for atrial fibrillation, prior to surgery, reversal of anticoagulation is with administration of vitamin K and fresh frozen plasma. If the patient had been receiving heparin, then only vitamin K is necessary as a reversal agent. For those on antiplatelet medications, such as clopidogrel and aspirin, platelets are often administered.

166. C: If a 76-year-old patient with a severe head injury has a history of 5 visits to the emergency department over the previous 18 months for minor to moderate injuries (cuts, fractures, bruising), bruises in various stages of heeling, and the patient's appearance is unkempt, and the patient is very thin (suggesting negligent care), the trauma nurse should suspect elder abuse. The appropriate authorities, such as Social Services or Adult Protective Services should be notified.

167. B: If a patient involved in a motor vehicle accident has typical lap-belt contusions (lap belt sign) and fracture of a lumbar vertebrae, the internal structure that is primarily at risk of contusion or transection is the pancreas. In addition, the patient may experience intestinal rupture. If only the lap belt contusions are present but not a lumbar fracture, then the risk is for intestinal rupture and/or mesenteric tear or contusion.

168. B: Ipsilateral neck pain, headache, ecchymosis and swelling of the neck, and ptosis with miosis (partial Horner syndrome) are consistent with traumatic carotid dissection, which may occur from direct neck trauma or hyperextension or rotation injuries. Other symptoms include hemiparesis, cervical bruit, and epistaxis. Carotid dissection may result in hematoma (intramural) or dilatation, which can lead to emboli and ischemic stroke. Dissection may be intra- or extracranial (most frequent) and may be spontaneous or trauma-related.

169. D: Only the intraventricular catheter allows for CSF drainage and sampling, but it is the most invasive device and increases risk of infection and complications, such as CSF leakage. However, it is also the most accurate and allows for instillation of contrast if necessary. The transducer must be leveled at the foramen of Monro and all ICP measurements done with the transducer at that level. The subdural/epidural catheter is the least invasive monitoring device although baseline drift occurs over time, reducing reliability.

170. A: Traumatic rupture of the aorta (a tear in the wall of the aorta contained by arterial adventitia and parietal pleura) may result from rapid deceleration, such as occurs with a fall from a large height or high impact motor vehicle accident. Although some patients are initially asymptomatic, some may complain of chest pain and/or pain in the posterior scapula area. Asymmetry of blood pressure in the upper extremities and widened pulse pressure are typical findings. The most common finding on a chest x-ray is a widened mediastinum (>8cm).

171. B: If a pregnant patient dies from traumatic injuries at 34 weeks (≥26 weeks) of gestation and the patient is provided continuous CPR, perimortem Cesarean to save the fetus must be carried out within 15 minutes. The neonate must be managed in the NICU, especially if it is many weeks premature. The Cesarean is done with a midline incision to most quickly access the fetus. The fetus is at risk for hypoxia and associated complications.

172. C: If a 76-year-old female patient who has generally been in good health has suffered a pathological fracture of the proximal femur while walking, resulting in a fall, the most likely cause is osteoporosis. All women age 65 and older should be routinely screened for osteoporosis. Bone loss often exceeds 35% before the patient experiences symptoms. The DEXA scan is the imaging method of choice with results expressed as T scores. A T score of minus 2 (-2) is diagnostic of osteoporosis and indicates bone mass is 20% less than normal.

173. A: If a dying patient tells the nurse that she sees her mother, who has been deceased for many years, the most appropriate response is: "Does seeing your mother comfort or frighten you?" Patients who are dying often report visits from loved ones who are deceased or from spiritual figures, such as angels or devils. The trauma nurse should neither challenge or support these perceptions but should encourage the patient to discuss feelings about them if the patient is still able to verbalize.

174. D: If a patient has spinal cord injury resulting from a gunshot wound, reflex testing for L4 injury is carried out at the knee. Reflex testing:

- C5 injury: Testing of biceps area, jaw jerk, and deltoid.
- C7 injury: Testing of triceps.
- T9 to T12 injury: Testing of pectoral, superficial abdominal.
- L4 injury: Testing of brachioradialis, knee.
- S1 injury: Testing of ankle.
- S3 to S4 injury: Testing of bulbo- or clitorocavernositis.
- S5 injury: Testing of anal wink.

175. B: To evaluate the function of cranial nerve XI (spinal accessory) for a patient with a traumatic neck injury, the trauma nurse should place hands on the patient's shoulders and ask the patient to shrug against resistance. Cranial nerve XI is especially at risk of injury with trauma to the neck, including whiplash injury, as well as cervical fractures and spinal cord injuries. Patients may complain of pain in the shoulder and exhibit weakness of the trapezius muscle.

Thank You

We at Mometrix would like to extend our heartfelt thanks to you, our friend and patron, for allowing us to play a part in your journey. It is a privilege to serve people from all walks of life who are unified in their commitment to building the best future they can for themselves.

The preparation you devote to these important testing milestones may be the most valuable educational opportunity you have for making a real difference in your life. We encourage you to put your heart into it—that feeling of succeeding, overcoming, and yes, conquering will be well worth the hours you've invested.

We want to hear your story, your struggles and your successes, and if you see any opportunities for us to improve our materials so we can help others even more effectively in the future, please share that with us as well. **The team at Mometrix would be absolutely thrilled to hear from you!** So please, send us an email (support@mometrix.com) and let's stay in touch.

> **If you'd like some additional help, check out these other resources we offer for your exam: http://MometrixFlashcards.com/TCRN**

Additional Bonus Material

Due to our efforts to try to keep this book to a manageable length, we've created a link that will give you access to all of your additional bonus material:

mometrix.com/bonus948/traumacrn